Overcoming Disabilities Despair:

9 steps for talking away what's getting you down.

Michael D. LeBow Ph.D., C. Psych.

Science & Humanities Press
Chesterfield Missouri

Copyright Notice:

Overcoming Disabilities Despair is copyright 2010 by Michael D. LeBow with all rights reserved.
Figures and photographs used for the cover are primarily derived objects in the Hemera Royalty Free collection, *the Big Box of Art*, assembled and modified with enhancement by Dr. Bud Banis

Publication Date, October, 2010
ISBN 9781596300637

Library of Congress Cataloging-in-Publication Data

LeBow, Michael D.
  Disabilities despair : 9 steps for talking away what's getting you down / Michael D. LeBow.
     p. cm.
  Includes bibliographical references and index.
  ISBN 978-1-59630-063-7 (alk. paper)
 1. People with disabilities--Mental health. 2. Cognitive therapy I. Title.
  RC451.4.H35L43 2010
  617'.0691425--dc22
                              2010032764

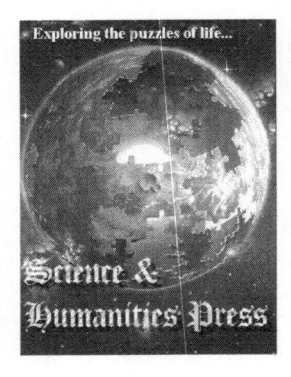

Science & Humanities Press
PO Box 7151
Chesterfield, MO 63006-7151
sciencehumanitiespress.com

For Alina:

You'll always be my sweetheart,
even when you're no longer "just a keed"

Other Books by Michael LeBow:

Behaviour modification: A significant method in nursing practice.

Rational hospital psychiatry: The reactive environment

Approaches to modifying patient behaviour

If only I were thin.

Weight control: The behavioural strategies

Child obesity: A new frontier of behaviour therapy

The thin plan

Adult obesity therapy

Overweight children.

Overweight teenagers: Don't bear the burden alone

Dieters snake pit

Preface

I hate being disabled. It can make everyday tasks seem like giant hurdles. It can make past joys seem like they'll never be repeated. It can make others seem like naysayers and critics, doubting your capabilities, doubting your capacities, finding you odd, finding you ugly. Probably worst of all, it can make the future seem like an abyss that's slowly but surely sucking you in. So, I hate being disabled because it can make you feel helpless, joyless, worthless, hopeless. It can do some of or all this, if you let it.

IF YOU LET IT.

Two years ago I began a clinical-research project to show how not to let it, though I had myself been trying not to let it for many years before; multiple sclerosis has been my unwholesome, unwelcome, and unkind companion for decades. The project, focusing on MS but applicable to other disabling conditions, involved how to question and challenge the disability assumptions that cause many of the disabled so much psychological anguish. Its premise, emanating from Cognitive Behavior Therapy (CBT), is what you tell yourself about yourself affects how you feel about yourself. Overcoming Disabilities Despair echoes that premise.

The book, which relies on the principles and practices of CBT, distills the project's procedures into an algorithm that guides those despairing about their disabilities into thinking better to feel more upbeat and more hopeful. Its lessons reflect my training in CBT and the works of such scholars as Drs. Aaron Beck and David Burns who have developed and refined this therapeutic approach. I have applied their wisdom to the disability area hoping to improve the lives of those who struggle daily with disabilities despair generated by the unwarranted assumptions they hold about disability and what it means to their present and future well-being. The book describes those assumptions and what to do about them.

Overcoming Disabilities Despair is a little book with, I hope, a big pay off. Copy any of the forms inside that you need whenever you need them, and by all means let me know whether the book helps you. I value your criticisms, questions, and comments, so please e-mail them to me at the University of Manitoba [mlebow@cc.umanitoba.ca].

MDL

Winnipeg, September 2009

Table of Contents

CHAPTER 1: Disability Stinks 1

CHAPTER 2: Assumptions: Some Raise Us Up, Some Drive Us Down 7

CHAPTER 3 Disability Assumption 1: Disability Diminishes Worth 21

CHAPTER 4 Disability Assumption 2: Disability Ends Happiness 37

CHAPTER 5 Disability Assumption 3: Disability Means Ugly 55

CHAPTER 6 Disability Assumption 4: Disability Means Helpless. 69

CHAPTER 7 Disability assumption #5: Disability Means Hopeless 79

CHAPTER 8 Disability Fallout 91

CHAPTER 9 A Closer Look Inside Your CBT Toolbox 103

LAST WORD: 115

REFERENCES 119

APPENDIX 1 121

APPENDIX 2 129

APPENDIX 3 133

APPENDIX 4 135

INDEX 137

CHAPTER 1: Disability Stinks

My right hand throbbed. The squeezing-pounding wouldn't stop.

My pen dropped. I swore for about 20 seconds. It was during the morning on a weekday early in June 1981, and I had just penned a page of psychobabble for a book I was doing when the pain began. As I sat in my cubbyhole office at the University where I teach, I wondered if this was a prelude to a worse agony. Downhill from 40 on?

I couldn't answer, but took solace in knowing that just two months earlier I'd run a marathon, even though finishing 2314 out of a pack of not too many more than that—and even though disappointing my eight-year-old son who thought I should have done better. For two weeks, each time I started to write the pain returned causing my productivity to drop, and as ridiculous as it sounds, I hated that slide in the pages-done-count the most. Actually, it was a fear of falling productivity that prompted me to call my family doctor. He knew what was wrong, I think, but believing I couldn't handle his diagnosis said nothing except, "I want Dr.—to look at this." That did scare me, somewhat.

Three weeks later I sat in a broom-closet of a room naked under a rapidly shredding paper robe waiting for a renowned specialist, who it turned out possessed the demeanor of Attila the Hun. Flanked by three male med-students, each one fresh enough to have only recently mastered the art of shaving, and two female also adolescent-looking want-to-be doctors, the guru had me do a heel-to-toe across the room. My exposed body shivered as he gleefully alerted his young followers that they were seeing MS in its early stages. The man seemed oblivious to the fact that I could hear and think. I now was too scared to be humiliated.

Two months later, after numbers of tests and unreturned phone calls from another white-coated-insensitive, I was told, "Don't go into a blue-funk. You have chronic progressive multiple sclerosis."

And so my journey into disability began. It took me years to understand what disability really means and the importance of trying to replenish the confidence, esteem, and power it so ruthlessly siphons.

PRESENT DAY

I love dining out—nicer the restaurant and better the food, greater the pleasure. Recently my wife and I treated ourselves to a posh, pricy palace of sumptuous cuisine. I didn't check the restrooms first, usually do; handicap accessibility is essential. But for the last few months, I had been getting through dinners undisturbed by that call of nature. Sadly, however, my luck ended halfway through this fancy meal.

I knew generally where the restroom was but nothing of its size or layout. Soon, though, I was to learn that there were two doors protecting its inner sanctum and, most disconcerting, that each doorway was smaller than the width of my walker. As I approached where I had to get, I could see that there might be a problem, but because my needs were great, I pushed through anyway. Bad decision. Like Winnie-the-Pooh— though not greedy, just needy--- I got stuck.

Immediately, a hot surge of panic began to course through me. If I didn't reach my objective soon—very soon, very very soon—someone, everyone, would see me pee-stained---Professor Peestained. Frantically I pushed and pulled. Nothing happened. Still stuck. And nature was really calling, and fear was really rising. Was this a W.C. Fields skit? I wasn't laughing. Luckily a short, strong guy with a, I suspect, similar urge, but without the fear I had, arrived. He easily freed my walker. Back to problem one; I still had to get into the inner room, a fact he sensed. He carefully angled my walker into the first room while I clutched the door-jam. Then he angled it into the main room, which had one urinal and one toilet. No way could I get my walker into the sit-down cubicle, undoubtedly engineered for agile Lilliputians, so he chose it and let me struggle with the one step-up urinal, which I negotiated successfully. He waited for me and freed me from the two rooms. A nice guy. I thanked him profusely.

As I returned to my table, my spirits nosedived. Why?

Overcoming Disabilities despair

Another example, not an uncommon one either as the similar incident in Chapter 3 suggests. I was at a mall and, for the first time in weeks, having a good time. On the mend from a recently broken arm, I couldn't steer my walker, so to get around I was using a wheelchair; my wife was pushing. Packed with shoppers, the mall was tricky to navigate. A kindly man of about 50 cornered us and to my wife said, "Is he having a good time?" Then, pointing to an open area a few feet ahead added, "If you want to park him right here and do some shopping, I'll watch him." Again, my up-spirits tumbled. Why?

MS AND MOOD

Likely when the Samaritan at the fancy restaurant freed me and the kindly gentleman at the mall spoke of me not to me and offered to park me and watch me, I said something to myself. And what I said each time triggered each emotional low. I'm not unique in having this happen, for in addition to sometimes feeling resentful, angry, or anxious, many disabled men and women regularly undergo drops in mood — some brief, some extended.

How far down-in-the-dumps are you? Do you believe that you cannot influence your disability? Do you believe that you burden loved-ones, that life is hopeless, that you are helpless? Do you spend hours a day saddened by what you cannot do? Do you find that you begin the day okay, but then something happens — someone says something or you read an article in the paper or you think about how things now are, how they were, how they will be — and your mood nosedives? Perhaps you then want to climb into bed and stay there. Or perhaps you descend to a level where you get through the day, but that's all — there's no joy. Possibly you cry a lot. Possibly you don't cry yet want to and can't. Possibly you feel such a profound sense of sadness and emptiness that you are depressed.

Different persons feel depression differently and to different degrees and will when depressed experience one or more of these:

- Sadness: feeling dispirited to despair to utter hopelessness

3

- Anhedonia: little or nothing pleases or interests
- Feeling worthless, guilty, empty
- Sleep problems: taking hours to fall asleep, waking up early and being unable to fall back asleep, or sleeping excessively
- Fatigue
- Little or no motivation
- Difficulty concentrating
- Indecisive, even about little things
- No appetite or nonstop eating and gaining
- Self-denigration

Suicidal thoughts: sometimes to the severely depressed person, ending life seems to be the only way to end mental pain. If you have such thoughts, seek help from a professional counsellor immediately. Go to the nearest free clinic or emergency hospital. Call a suicide hotline. Don't wait. Act right away.

LESS MOPING, MORE COPING

To feel better—happier, more alive, stronger, more fulfilled—stop drowning in the knowledge you're disabled. By providing you with a few critical swimming lessons, this book will try to help you. It will show you how to:

- activate and find the pleasure and mastery that activation brings—inactivity and the blues share a bed.
- stand-up for your rights
- be more hopeful and upbeat about the present and future
- look for more positives in your world

- be more helpful to yourself and those who help you
- communicate better with friends and family
- communicate better with yourself
- feel more empowered
- be flexible instead of rigid when evaluating yourself — see the shades of gray and not just blacks or whites
- become, in Dr. Stephen Covey's words from *The 7 habits of highly effective people*, less reactive and more pro-active.

A tall order. To fill it, you'll practice a set of feel-better strategies that I use in my own skirmishes with the despair of being disabled — disabilities despair. Some zero-in on actions, others on thinking. When applied with patience, perseverance, and courage, they promise to help — and they don't require pills to do so.

Those targeting thinking belong, for the most part, to a school of mood therapy known as Cognitive Behavior Therapy (CBT). Developed during the 1960s by Drs. Albert Ellis and Aaron Beck, working independently, CBT is popular and effective; this manual borrows mostly from Beck and his student, Dr. David Burns. The Ellis and Beck approaches differ from one another in several ways, but for both of them a major guiding principle is: you feel bad largely because of what you tell yourself.

Negative thoughts — negative moods. A depressed man encounters his female neighbor who asks how he's doing. The man says, "Not so well," and because the lady grimaces, he thinks, This gal believes I'm a complaining-loser. He doesn't really know what is bothering her, if indeed anything is, but nonetheless concludes the worst. Or, suppose a somewhat despondent woman with rheumatoid arthritis (RA), who now needs a walker, accepts an invitation to spend an evening at a local fancy restaurant. However, she soon has second thoughts about going and considers backing out because she worries that she'll be unable to lift herself from the restaurant's deep chair; RA has substantially weakened her. But she does go and when finished manages to rise successfully. Time for a mental pat on the back, yet she denies herself this. Instead she thinks, This is only what people should be able to do. Or, for another instance of living in the negative, let's say she misses a subordinate's accounting error, costing her company several hundred dollars. Understandably, she feels bad. But instead of resolving to be more vigilant next time and taking steps to backup her resolve, she reasons, What's just happened to me, like all the crap in my life, is my destiny. CBT therapists would help her and similarly depressed and dispirited individuals uncover and eliminate such ways of thinking.

They arise, as do many other despair-generating thoughts, from rigid and stifling maladaptive assumptions some people hold about life and the way things should be. Examples include:

I should always succeed

I should always be happy

I should always be approved of

I should never make a mistake

Often the individual doesn't even know that he or she buys into such dysfunctional assumptions. They remain hidden until some unpleasant experience such as a setback, an ambiguous glance, snub or comment from another, or an error of some sort summons them from their dark places. Hidden assumptions are ruthless, and there are many of them. They are so unreasonable, so impossible, that they are guaranteed to make the person trying to live up to them feel bad.

You'll read about a special kind of dysfunctional assumption, the disability-assumption, that even if not hidden is always ruthless. We will identify five such disability assumptions. They take an If... then form such as, if I'm disabled, then I can never be happy again, and there's nothing I can do about it. The disability assumptions will make you hurt because they shout game-over, no hope, no chance to cope or be happy or be valued. You'll learn more about these unforgiving misery-makers next and then in later chapters what to do about them.

Overcoming Disabilities despair

CHAPTER 2: Assumptions: Some Raise Us Up, Some Drive Us Down

When I was in grammar school, my physical education teacher, coach of all the school's athletics, was also my math teacher. At the time, he was a V-shape who wore his shirt two buttons open at the top. He really believed that if you weren't a good athlete you couldn't be very good at anything male. He never actually said that, but his actions nonetheless shouted it: he bought doughnuts and other treats for the good athletes, not the so-so ones; he huddled with the good athletes, not the so-so ones; he shared jokes and personal stories with the good athletes, not the so-so ones. And he literally shunned the brightest of the budding mathematicians who couldn't with even moderate proficiency kick footballs, dribble basketballs, or catch fly balls. As well, he ignored those few boys who preferred the chessboard and camera to anything sports, and viciously ridiculed those very few boys who, God help them, were fat.

This misguided educator was clear about who in his eyes was worthy and, because to us was the epitome, the model man to emulate, who should be worthy in our eyes, also. In grade eight most boys and many girls echoed coach's axioms: good athlete, worthy guy; bad athlete, unworthy guy.

Hard rules to live by. We judged our male peers by them, however, and sadly for those of us who never made it as jocks but desperately wished we had, ourselves, too. Turning such rules inward and giving them high standing in your personal code for life could be devastating, for it put too much on the line by implying: "If I'm not a good athlete, I'm unworthy" — which isn't far from, "If I'm not a good athlete, I'm worthless." Thinking that way, I did, was a slippery-slope into despair even depression. When I couldn't make the A-team in basketball and failed Little League tryouts in baseball, I went beyond reasoning that possibly sports was not my forte: I attacked my self-worth.

And that hurt. For most of us such assumptions, though hidden from consciousness until activated, eventually will cause unremitting pain. Because unpleasant assumptions lie quietly out of awareness until activated, at least most of them do, cognitive behavior therapists like Dr. David Burns, author of *The feeling good handbook*, call them silent assumptions.

Their silence is only temporary, however, for once triggered they get loud and can then take control of our moods, propelling us into depression, guilt, discouragement, insecurity, or any number of unpleasant feelings. Here's what might happen say cognitive therapists Dr. Aaron Beck and colleagues in their classic, *Cognitive therapy of depression:*

1) Something happens that brings into focus a sensitive area:
   "John doesn't approve of how I spent the money."

2) A dysfunctional assumption—rule to live by---lurking below the level of awareness is triggered:
   "I must have approval to be happy."

3) Conclusion:
   "Now, I can't be happy."

4) Unpleasant emotion results:
   sadness, possibly depression

When I blew the tryout for the Little League team, my failure triggered the self-indictment, the self-defining assumption, "If I'm not a good athlete, I must be unworthy." I concluded, "I'm unworthy." As a result, I felt downtrodden and inferior and in many ways for years afterwards found confirmation of this scurrilous indictment.

Certainly not all the assumption-rules that guide us generate misery. Productive assumptions, many inculcated in us directly or indirectly by our parents and teachers and peers, help us persevere, excel, choose right over wrong, and live enabling, satisfying lives. Bill Porter, the door-to-door Portland salesman disabled from birth by cerebral palsy owes much of his high functioning to his mother who explicitly taught him that patience and persistence yielded success. More than not, productive assumption-rules are flexible, positive, self-improving, and happiness-promoting.

Destructive ones, in contrast, often phrased as "if-then's" and frequently laced with "shoulds", "musts", and "oughts" between the "if's-then's" are rigid, punitive, self-effacing, and self-defeating. They saddle us with impossibles like these:

"If I'm not thin, I can't be happy"

"I should be strong to be a man"

"If I'm not beautiful, I'm not valuable"

"I should look handsome everyday"

"I must have approval to be happy"

"I must always be successful"

"If I'm flawed in any way, people won't accept me"

"I must always be accepted to be worthy"

"If I'm heavy, I have no will power"

"If I'm heavy, I can't be happy"

"If I'm heavy, there's nothing I like about me"

"If I'm heavy, I should hide"

"If I'm heavy, I have no sex appeal"

"If I'm heavy, I'm ugly"

(...)

Once activated by an event illuminating a sensitive area of our lives, such as a perceived vulnerability---an Achilles' heel—the destructive assumptions will distort thoughts to ruin moods. To many of the disabled, there is no area more sensitive, no vulnerability more sensed, than their disability, per se.

Probably beginning with the trauma of hearing that a disabling condition like multiple sclerosis or rheumatoid arthritis is to be your life's companion or realizing that the accident you've recently suffered has crippled you in some way, you've become hypersensitive to anything you'll hear or see having to do with being disabled. You've been sensitized to disability, and such magnified sensitivity makes you easy prey for one or more of the disability assumptions that follow.

FIVE DISABILITY ASSUMPTIONS

Each in its own way addresses what your being disabled leads you to assume about yourself. Possibly what you assume is that others overlook and devalue you as a person. Or possibly what you assume is that because you need a wheelchair, walker, or cane, others judge you as less competent. Maybe what you assume is that you are helpless, that your opportunities for enjoyment and independence are few, or that your future is hopeless. If you assume any of these or similar nasties, you are a candidate for feeling resentful, discouraged, inadequate, inferior, or frankly depressed. The disability assumptions suck-dry self-esteem, self-confidence, feelings of well-being, happiness, and zest for living.

Those I name next—maybe you're able to name others—are snakes in hiding but lurking nearby, ready to strike and poison your mind and mood. Here are the most venomous five and how you express them to yourself:

If I'm Disabled, My Worth is Diminished, and There's Nothing I Can Do About It

Feeling worthy is the center of self-esteem. Feeling otherwise is a knife in the heart. Signs that you maybe assuming that being disabled diminishes worth include believing disability makes you easy to ignore or take for granted, pitiable, and inferior in the sense of incompetent or significantly less competent.

I used to assume that disability and capability could not coexist in

the same body. Until I began really listening to my inner voice when feeling down, I didn't know I assumed that about myself. My inner voice was whispering, MS has stolen so much from you, you're no longer as effective as you should be, and there's nothing you can do about it. These days I still hear that voice, but when it intrudes, I shut-it-up in ways I'll explain in future chapters. A friend with MS, who also assumes that disability diminishes worth, ties worth to unwanted pity.

As said, different people may express this assumption differently, but the essence of it is always the same: disability diminishes worth. Likewise with the other disability assumptions, different people may express them differently and one person may express even the same assumption differently in different circumstances. Nonetheless, the essence of each assumption aroused never varies.

If I'm Disabled, I Can Never Be Happy Again, and There's Nothing I Can Do About It

Life's fun times, heartfelt pleasures, and successes come in many different packages. Watching a movie with friends, seeing your child's first soccer goal, writing a letter to the editor of the city's major newspaper, dining with your lover at a fancy restaurant, reading and understanding a difficult chemistry book, authoring a short-story, hearing the boss praise your efforts, solving a perplexing computer problem — the possibilities are endless. If your inner voice proclaims that because you now have a disabling condition, life holds no promise now or in the future of similar pleasures and triumphs, you'll likely avoid opportunities to experience them.

If I'm Disabled, I'm Ugly, and There's Nothing I Can Do About It

Expressions of this assumption include avoiding situations of intimacy because you believe yourself to be unappealing, misinterpreting the looks of others as indications that you appear strange, thinking that others are uncomfortable if near you, and shunning efforts to dress well, groom, or otherwise look better.

If I'm Disabled, I'm Helpless, and There's Nothing I Can Do About It

The helplessness assumption can be expressed in many ways,

including but not limited to:

believing that because you are disabled almost everything is now beyond your abilities to control

believing that because you are disabled, you can no longer protect yourself or your family believing that because you are disabled, you burden your family and friends.

The list of possibilities is extensive.

If I'm Disabled, I Have No Hope for the Future, and There's Nothing I Can Do About It

Some disabled folks equate having a worsening disabling condition like rheumatoid arthritis or multiple sclerosis to living under the fabled Sword of Damocles. I'm guilty of doing that, sometimes. To me, MS overpowers. It threatens. It waits. It terrorizes and the fear breeds feelings of futility and hopelessness. Like the last ghost to visit Scrooge, the hopelessness assumption is the most frightening. It gazes into the unknown and forecasts inescapable, unchangeable doom and gloom. The hopelessness assumption fosters pessimism and cynicism. And that's dangerous, for pessimism and cynicism will make you want to quit trying to do better and to stop planning for the future. Such feelings only bring the merciless sword closer.

Thankfully, feeling that everything is hopeless does not mean that everything is hopeless. Feeling that there is every reason to give-up does not mean that there is every reason to give-up. Feeling that life is going straight into the dumper does not mean that life is going straight into the dumper. Feeling a certain way does not mean, argues Dr. Burns, that things are in fact that way. To believe otherwise, to believe that feelings are certainties, is a cognitive error he terms emotional reasoning. It promotes giving-up and giving-in and leaves you continually moping and rarely coping. I'll have more to say about the problems of reasoning from emotions and, most important, what to do instead.

Misery-generating assumptions can be triggered as said when something happens that shouts you are disabled; possibly several nasty assumptions activate at the same time when the trigger is pulled. No matter how many assumptions are aroused, however, the result is almost certainly going to be despair. If that's what's happening to you, perhaps there is some solace in knowing that you're not alone. Many of the thousands upon thousands of disabled individuals in this world suffer recurrent and devastating drops in mood because of what they assume their disabilities mean to their lives now and in the future.

Overcoming Disabilities despair

What they suffer from is disabilities despair.

This book is about disabilities despair and how to rid yourself of it. In five of the eight chapters that follow, you'll see examples of disabilities despair and what people with conditions similar to yours do to stop it in order to feel better about themselves, their world, and their future. You'll learn how to identify what you tell yourself—think—before feeling dispirited and then how to uncover the misery-making assumptions getting you down, which are behind the self talk. As you have seen, not only do these assumptions forecast dire consequences, they also deny possible solutions. Your task will be to locate each despair-causing assumption and then, by questioning its nasty predictions and challenging its denial of solutions, to dispute its truth. To be nicer to yourself, to feel better about yourself, and to act better toward yourself, battle both parts of each assumption affecting you.

So, in the chapters that follow, you're going to become an assiduous inner-directed and inner-focused mind detective—a Hercules Poirot—who hunts down despair and gets rid of it by tracking down thoughts to uncover, question, and challenge and ultimately dispute misery-making assumptions. Although the nine step algorithm chapters 3 through 7 describe and exemplify is simple and straightforward, it's no quick-fix. This mood-lifting program requires time, patience, practice, and perseverance to work, but by making you a care-provider instead of a care-receiver, active instead of passive, it empowers. And by helping you build skills needed to handle the setbacks that inevitably happen, it's future oriented.

Before reading the mood-lifting chapters, however, I suggest you take the Assumptions of Disability Inventory that follows and plan to retake it periodically, especially when you're ready to apply the book's procedures to yourself.

Overcoming Disabilities despair

LeBOW ASSUMPTIONS OF DISABILITY INVENTORY

This inventory is primarily for those who are disabled, especially those disabled to the extent they require a cane, walker, or wheelchair.

DESCRIPTION AND INSTRUCTIONS:

The inventory comprises 31 statements that reflect your opinions about your being disabled. Each asks you to judge, from "Not At All" to "A Lot," the extent you agree with the statement. Total scores will vary from 0 (if you answered "Not At All" to each of them) to 93 (if you answered "A Lot" to each of them). The lower your total score the better, meaning the greater your freedom from debilitating disability assumptions.

Take the inventory now and retake it periodically as you learn to question and challenge the misery-generating disability assumptions depressing you. By retaking it as you try out the book's procedures, you'll be able to judge (as your total score lowers) how much you are improving. As well, you'll be able to judge, as regards each particular statement, how your ratings change. Your objective is to move from individual statement-ratings of 3 and 2 ("A Lot" and "Moderately") to those of 1 and 0 ("Somewhat" and "Not At All"). A recording sheet for your benefit follows the questionnaire.

1. Because I am disabled, I've lost most chances to enjoy life. To what extent do you agree?

0 (Not At All) 1 (Somewhat) 2 (Moderately) 3 (A Lot)

2. Because I am disabled, I no longer have anything to offer others. To what extent do you agree?

0 (Not At All) 1 (Somewhat) 2 (Moderately) 3 (A Lot)

3. Because I am disabled, I burden friends. To what extent do you agree?

0 (Not At All) 1 (Somewhat) 2 (Moderately) 3 (A Lot)

Overcoming Disabilities despair

4. Because I am disabled, others who are not disabled are uncomfortable around me. To what extent do you agree?

0 (Not At All) 1 (Somewhat) 2 (Moderately) 3 (A Lot)

5. Because I am disabled, I am less worthy. To what extent do you agree?

0 (Not At All) 1 (Somewhat) 2 (Moderately) 3 (A Lot)

6. Because I am disabled, I have less to offer others. To what extent do you agree?

0 (Not At All) 1 (Somewhat) 2 (Moderately) 3 (A Lot)

7. Because I am disabled, I am less socially appealing. To what extent do you agree?

0 (Not At All) 1 (Somewhat) 2 (Moderately) 3 (A Lot)

8. Others don't accept me as their equal now that I am disabled. To what extent do you agree.

0 (Not At All) 1 (Somewhat) 2 (Moderately) 3 (A Lot)

9. Because I am disabled, all the changes in my life will be negative. To what extent do you agree?

0 (Not At All) 1 (Somewhat) 2 (Moderately) 3 (A Lot)

10. Because I am disabled, I'm easier to ignore. To what extent do you agree?

0 (Not At All) 1 (Somewhat) 2 (Moderately) 3 (A Lot)

11. Because I am disabled, I'm ugly. To what extent do you agree?

0 (Not At All) 1 (Somewhat) 2 (Moderately) 3 (A Lot)

12. Because I am disabled, there is little I can do about the problems facing me. To what extent you agree?

0 (Not At All) 1 (Somewhat) 2 (Moderately) 3 (A Lot)

13. Because I am disabled, I have little or no chance of doing something in the future I can be proud of. To what extent do you agree?

0 (Not At All) 1 (Somewhat) 2 (Moderately) 3 (A Lot)

14. Because I am disabled. To what extent do you agree?

0 (Not At All) 1 (Somewhat) 2 (Moderately) 3 (A Lot)

15. Because I am disabled, most of the future changes in my life will likely be negative. To what extent do you agree?

0 (Not At All) 1 (Somewhat) 2 (Moderately) 3 (A Lot)

16. Because I am disabled, I'm no longer able to do the important things. To what extent do you agree?

0 (Not At All) 1 (Somewhat) 2 (Moderately) 3 (A Lot)

17. Because I am disabled, most others pity me. To what extent do you agree?

0 (Not At All) 1 (Somewhat) 2 (Moderately) 3 (A Lot)

18. Because I am disabled, my future looks hopeless. To what extent do you agree?

0 (Not At All) 1 (Somewhat) 2 (Moderately) 3 (A Lot)

19. Because I am disabled, I burden my family. To what extent do you agree?

0 (Not At All) 1 (Somewhat) 2 (Moderately) 3 (A Lot)

20. Because I am disabled, life no longer is fun and exciting. To what extent do you agree?

0 (Not At All) 1 (Somewhat) 2 (Moderately) 3 (A Lot)

21. Now that I am disabled, I am vulnerable. To what extent do you agree?

0 (Not At All) 1 (Somewhat) 2 (Moderately) 3 (A Lot)

Overcoming Disabilities despair

22. If I can't do as much as I used to, I'm not as worthy as I once was. To what extent do you agree?

0 (Not At All) 1 (Somewhat) 2 (Moderately) 3 (A Lot)

23. Because I am disabled, I'm less appealing sexually. To what extent do you agree?

0 (Not At All) 1 (Somewhat) 2 (Moderately) 3 (A Lot)

24. Because I am disabled, I have little chance in the future of excelling. To what extent do you agree?

0 (Not At All) 1 (Somewhat) 2 (Moderately) 3 (A Lot)

25. To many others, my disability is like a neon sign flashing avoid me. To what extent do you agree?

0 (Not At All) 1 (Somewhat) 2 (Moderately) 3 (A Lot)

26. Because I am disabled, I've lost all chances to enjoy life. To what extent do you agree?

0 (Not At All) 1 (Somewhat) 2 (Moderately) 3 (A Lot)

27. Because I am disabled, I have much less to offer others. To what extent do you agree?

0 (Not At All) 1 (Somewhat) 2 (Moderately) 3 (A Lot)

28. Because I am disabled, all future changes in my life will likely be negative. To what extent do you agree?

0 (Not At All) 1 (Somewhat) 2 (Moderately) 3 (A Lot)

29. Because I am disabled, more people than ever before do not wish to be around me. To what extent do you agree?

0 (Not At All) 1 (Somewhat) 2 (Moderately) 3 (A Lot)

30. There is little I can do about the problems my being disabled causes me. To what extent do you agree?

0 (Not At All) 1 (Somewhat) 2 (Moderately) 3 (A Lot)

Overcoming Disabilities despair

31. Because I am disabled, I'm unappealing sexually. To what extent do you agree?

0 (Not At All) 1 (Somewhat) 2 (Moderately) 3 (A Lot)

TOTAL SCORE=

Overcoming Disabilities despair

ANSWER SHEET Record your answers to the inventory each time you take it by putting a 0(not at all), 1(somewhat), 2(moderately), or 3(a lot) in the space to the right of the numbers, each of which represents one of the 31 statements. Then, total your score (T) and indicate the date (D).

	time1	time 2	time 3	time 4
1				
2				
3				
4				
5				
6				
7				
8				
9				
10				
11				
12				
13				
14				
15				

Overcoming Disabilities despair

16				
17				
18				
19				
20				
21				
22				
23				
24				
25				
26				
26				
27				
29				
30				
31				
Total				
Date				

CHAPTER 3 Disability Assumption 1: Disability Diminishes Worth

Afflicted with multiple sclerosis at the age of 33, Julie Anne Jonah sufferers intermittent bouts of despair mainly because of what she assumes being disabled means to her life. This chapter describes her case and how, using the multi-step algorithm, she begins to conquer this despair.

Algorithm Overview

How do you give-up a dysfunctional assumption, so ingrained that likely you don't even know it's there? That's exactly what the algorithm shows you how to do. Relying upon the principles and practices found in cognitive and behavioral sciences, the algorithm helps you identify, question, and challenge disability assumptions. Step by step, Julie and those individuals described in chapters 4-7 apply this system to mitigate their disabilities despair. With soul-searching and self-monitoring, they accomplish this task by asking and answering these critical questions:

1) What upset me?
2) How do I feel?
3) How upset am I?
4) What am I assuming (telling myself)?
5) How strongly do I believe what I'm assuming is really true?
6) Is the assumption I'm making logical, fair, or true?
7) How can I argue against the assumption bringing me down?
8) What sorts of questions should I ask myself to

argue against it?

9) How can I prove to myself that I can do what the assumption says I can't do?

10) Could I have interpreted things differently, not become upset?

11) Have I changed my mind about how true the assumption is?

12) Have I changed my mind about how I feel about what initially upset me?

About Julie and MS

For years, MS has been Julie's foe, and for years many things have put it in her face. Most waking hours, were she to color her moods, she would rapidly run out of grays and blacks, certainly faster than any other color, for Julie like so many with MS, has disabilities despair.

MS is a disease of the brain and spinal cord---the central nervous system — and is the most common neurological dysfunction afflicting young adults, mostly women but men often more severely. Ages of onset are usually from 15 to 50 years, yet there are reports of younger individuals having it. MS occurs more often in Caucasians having Northern Europe ancestry and in those living farther from the Equator, be it North or South of it.

MS is a demyelinating disease, meaning that the fatty material covering nerves, deteriorates. When the myelin goes, so does coordinated, quick, and efficient movement. This happens because myelin, think of it as insulation like on an electric cable, allows the nerves it shields to send and receive impulses without interference. Suppose you want to push your chair away from the kitchen table and stand up. Before demyelination, no problem. You did them easily and speedily with hardly a thought. After demyelination, big problem. The nerves involved in those acts have been stripped of their covering, so you struggle or simply can't do them. Quick flowing movement has slowed, become confused, or impossible.

Overcoming Disabilities despair

What causes demyelination? Believe it or not, you probably do. The culprit, some scientists think, is the MS sufferer's immune system when its soldiers—T-cells, killer cells, and hungry macrophages resembling amoebas —attack and inflame the myelin. In time, scar tissue forms where myelin once was. MS destroys the best friend relationship, the normal relationship, between you and your immune system, but no one knows exactly why or how. The best guess is that an wholesome alliance forms between a gene or genes and some pathogen in the environment, a virus perhaps, that commands these soldiers to rebel against and attack the central nervous system. But no one knows for sure.

This how and why MS mystery is not nearly as disconcerting to MS victims as the what-to-do and expect MS mystery. Simply put, the disease is untreatable and unpredictable and its course inexact: some MS victims are disabled immediately; some not for years; some never; some go through relapsing-remitting phases with flare-ups and recoveries, the most typical kind of MS, and then, not all but many, will begin a secondary phase of progressive deterioration; and some, like Julie, will deteriorate slowly and steadily from onset. Abilities and functions compromised include but are not limited to walking, seeing, speaking, standing, defecating, and urinating. Who will experience what and when during the illness can't be reliably forecast, but it's likely most sufferers will sometime when battling their disease have to face conspicuous, recurrent, debilitating fatigue, and over half of those who do will claim it's their worst problem.

Julie says it is her worst. She left her job, accepting her companies disability package, so she maintains, because of it. Julie and her husband, no children, are financially comfortable living on just his income. Nonetheless, she misses the six-figure salary being an advertising executive brought her. But, in truth, she misses the job's daily give and take even more. When she thinks about it, Julie realizes that fatigue was only part of the reason she left her career in advertising, and not even the most important part either. Loss of self-confidence played a larger role. She started doubting her abilities to live up to the job's demands, a doubt reinforced by her assumption that coworkers believed that ability and disability could not coexist for long in a hectic workplace. To Julie, her worth was diminishing. She started defining herself as disabled and losing sureness in who she was and could be. Thinking this way left her feeling dispirited and downtrodden.

To a significant extent, Julie's thoughts reflect disability assumption 1 — disability diminishes worth — and her despair results from it. When she can stop assuming that disability and worth are so inextricably entangled, she'll move closer to being able to lift her mood.

But one swallow does not make a summer. She'll need to dispute this assumption many times in different situations before it leaves her alone and she truly accepts that her competencies are not automatically or necessarily diminished by disability. Still even one small success in disputing disability assumption 1 is a very significant start on this very important journey. The following example of her laying waste to one instance of this assumption is that start.

Julie's written thoughts in the step-by-step example reveal how she persuades herself to doubt and then dispute disability assumption 1. (General instructions for completing each step precede her written comments.)

STEP 1 DESCRIBE WHAT HAPPENED THAT UPSET YOU

Something upset you. Write down what. Possibly nothing specific you can name took place other than just thinking of things — daydreams, recollections, worries about what's to come — and your despair seems to deepen. Write down your thoughts.

Julie writes, "Ever since the doctor told me I have MS, a good five years ago, I haven't had many happy days — fluctuate usually between feeling blah and feeling blue. Sometimes though I'm okay, like this afternoon. I wasn't thinking about being disabled and not working anymore. But that soon changed. Jacki and I were clothes-hunting at the mall. She doesn't mind pushing my wheelchair, thank God. If she did mind, I wouldn't go. It was really hot, and I was feeling kind of happy. Then this woman of I guess about 60 stopped where we were and looking only at Jacki throughout said, 'Is she enjoying herself? I'm glad that she has a chance to get out and see everything. She reminds me of Mom.'

Immediately I thought how ridiculous that sounds. How could I

Overcoming Disabilities despair

remind her of her mother. I'm even younger than she (the daughter) is. The woman just put years on me because I'm in a wheelchair.

Continuing with her description of her mother, the woman said, 'Mom, was chair bound her last 10 years and in a nursing home. I pushed her chair all over town. I do hope she's,' pointing at me without looking at me, 'having a good time today....'

I was, but after that woman talked, I felt really down."

STEP 2. NAME AND RATE YOUR NEGATIVE FEELINGS

Write down your feelings—name them—and rate how strongly from 1 (hardly at all) to 100 (extremely) you feel them.

After the interchange with the woman, Julie states and rates her feelings as follows:

despair (70)

anger (60)

STEP 3. IDENTIFY EACH MISERY-GENERATING ASSUMPTION TRIGGERED

Ask yourself why you feel the way you feel. To answer, try to recover the thoughts you had when the situation that upset you happened—replay your inner voice.

Julie writes, "I really don't know why I feel bad. That woman was only trying to be nice. I really think she meant well. Okay, I wasn't happy about being compared to her dear dead Mom, but that wasn't really the problem. When I think about it, what really got me was hearing myself referred to in the third person—SHE, SHE, SHE—as if, even with simple questions, I'm too decrepit to understand, too diminished to answer."

From those thoughts search for each misery-making assumption triggered.

The misery-generating assumption the passerby's words and actions triggered caused Julie's drop in spirit. If she doesn't know what assumption is responsible, she can find out by capturing her thoughts reflecting it, a practice in Burns' *The feeling good handbook* named, "the ." The vertical arrow technique is the powerful lens that reveals the hard to see parts of thoughts. With the vertical arrow technique, one analyzes one's thoughts, thought by thought. Each thought suggests a more basic one, and tracing each back to what it suggests or means gets to the root thought—the underlying disability assumption.

So, Julie has to ask herself when the woman spoke about me instead of to me what did I say to myself. Julie has to recall the woman's spoken words and then hear her own unspoken ones—her own thoughts. Julie has to eavesdrop on herself.

After doing this, Julie was able to write that her first thought was, "I look feeble in this wheelchair."

Then, Julie has to ask herself if that is true and I look feeble in the wheelchair, what is so upsetting about that? What does it mean?

After doing this, Julie was able to write that her second thought was, "Maybe it means I appear as if I've lost it, so why would she or anyone else want to talk to me now." Then asking herself if that were true what's so upsetting about it, and what does it mean, Julie could write, "Maybe it means I'm not worth her time and attention like I would be if I appeared normal, so ignoring me is easy."

Julie's Disabling Thoughts:

1) I look feeble in this wheelchair.

2) I probably appear as if I've lost it, so why would she or anyone else want to talk to me now.

3) I'm not worth her time and attention like I would be if I appeared normal, so ignoring me is easy.

Having uncovered the disabling thoughts, usually three is sufficient, Julie has to find the underlying disability assumption(s) making her unhappy.

Possible Disability Assumptions:

1) If I'm disabled, my worth is diminished, and there's nothing I can do about it

2) If I'm disabled, I can never be happy again, and

there's nothing I can do about it

3) If I'm disabled, I look ugly, and there's nothing I can do about it

4) If I'm disabled, I'm helpless, and there's nothing I can do about it

5) If I'm disabled, I have no hope for the future, and there's nothing I can do about it

After reviewing the list of possible disability assumptions, Julie writes,

"When I think about it, I guess the first assumption in the list of five is the one governing me to some degree, although all of them are probably a part of me now."

Disability Assumption Identified:

If I'm disabled, my worth is diminished (expressed in this situation as being easy to ignore or take for granted) and there's nothing I can do about it.

STEP 4. RATE HOW MUCH YOU AGREE THAT THE ASSUMPTION IDENTIFIED IS TRUE

For each assumption triggered, rate to what extent you agree that it is true using the scale that follows.

0. Not at all

1. Somewhat

2. Moderately

3. A Lot

Julie's rating: #3 A Lot

STEP 5. DISPUTE BY QUESTIONING THE ASSUMPTION IDENTIFIED

Question its value, logic, fairness, evidence, or accuracy, or all these qualities.

Overcoming Disabilities despair

Possible Questions to Ask:

1) What Are The Pluses of Accepting And Those of Rejecting The Assumption?
2) Would I Say it to Someone Else?
3) How Do I Figure?
4) Am I Thinking Rigidly?
5) Am I Labeling?
6) What Are The Exceptions (Search for Exceptions)?
7) Am I Fortune-telling?
8) Am I Catastrophizing?
9) Am I Letting My Feelings Be My Reality?
10) What Would a High-priced Lawyer Say?

Actual Questions Asked:

Question 1: What Are The Pluses of Accepting and Those of Rejecting The Assumption?

- Look closely at the assumption.
- What does accepting it do for you?
- What does rejecting it do for you?

Do the pluses of rejecting outnumber or outweigh, or both outnumber and outweigh, those of accepting?

If the pluses of rejecting are greater, likely they are, you have put into question the assumption's utility for you and by so doing siphoned a bit of its power over you.

Julie writes, "I can see no advantages to accepting the assumption that disability

diminishes my worth, but I can see advantages to it. For one thing, by rejecting it I'll be making a stand for better treatment, and I'll probably get better treatment; for another, I'll feel like I matter, and I like feeling that way better than feeling that I don't; and for yet

28

another, by rejecting the assumption and doing something constructive about people who treat me otherwise, I'll be making things easier and better for the next gal or guy in a wheelchair.

Thinking differently boosts both my self-esteem and that old power feeling I

used to have in advertising, the feeling that I'm still a force in this universe. I want that back."

Question 2: Would I Say it to Someone Else?

Harder on yourself than on others? If so, ask why the double standard, one for you and one for the rest of us, and the unfairness of what you're doing will cry out.

Julie writes,"I wouldn't tell someone in my position: Listen, I'm sorry, but now that everyone can see that you're disabled, you're no longer as worthy as the able people are. Able people will be more likely than ever before to overlook you. And rightly so. It's unfair for you to expect to be treated otherwise. They are in a superior class, so they'll talk down to you or just ignore you. That's just the way it is. Accept it.

Horrible. But that's kind of what I'm telling me, and it's unfair to have a double standard — one for others, one for me."

Question 3: How Do I Figure?

(A) Is the evidence for what you're telling yourself solid?

Julie writes, "The woman did indeed ignore me but that does not mean she did it because I'm in fact unworthy of her attention or because she believed that I'm unworthy of her attention. Also, there is no evidence that this sort of thing will happen again and again."

(B) Is what you're telling yourself logical?

Julie writes, "Does anyone have the power to determine another individual's worth? Am I really unworthy if somebody ignores me? If she doesn't pay attention to me , does that mean I'm unworthy? If she pays it , does that mean I'm worthy? The fact is her behavior neither proves nor disproves my worth. Suppose I had encountered four people in the mall, and let's say two ignored me and two didn't. What does that prove? Am I less worthy than the able are or as worthy as them? The point is that my worth is independent of how others treat me. The woman ignored me, that's for sure. But what she did or didn't do, what anyone does or doesn't do, can't determine my worth because it's not theirs to determine. It's not on the table. Others can hurt me or please me, but not prove or disprove my value. It's simply not within anyone's power to do that."

STEP 6 DISPUTE BY CHALLENGING THE ASSUMPTION IDENTIFIED

Dispute the assumption by challenging behaviorally the part that says, "and there's nothing I can do about it."

Possible Challenges to Make:

1) Challenge by Assertiveness

2) Challenge by Activation

3) Challenge by Problem-solving

4) Challenge by Contracting

5) Challenge by Relaxation

6) Challenge by Exposure

Actual Challenges Made:

Challenge 1: Challenge by Assertiveness

Act better towards yourself, feel better about yourself. Simple but true, though often difficult to carry out. To challenge, to lay waste to the second part of the assumption, the part that says you can do nothing about it, do something about it. Acting assertively, standing-up for your rights, is one of several challenges possible; it fits here well.

Julie could have communicated with the mall lady in one of three ways:

passively, aggressively, or assertively. The passive method is the say-nothing, say-little strategy. The woman talks, and Julie doesn't or does so very meekly: head down, eyes downcast, posture slumped.

Overcoming Disabilities despair

More than anything else, the passive way avoids trouble.

Not so the aggressive way. It jump-starts trouble by attempting to do to the woman what the woman has done to her, namely trample feelings, deny dignity. Julie could have said, but wisely didn't say, "Listen, I'm here and you're probably too stupid to see that. When you come across somebody in a wheelchair you idiot, don't ignore them. Don't let that happen again."

The aggressive way dominates and hurts and is thoughtless, pompous, and rude. Done angrily, loudly, quickly, threateningly, and glaringly (eyes blazing), it brings out the worst in everyone. For awhile the aggressor feels powerful, but the hapless target may want to or actually hit back or spit—probably will angrily and confusedly walk away and in the future ignore others in wheelchairs.

The Assertive way, the third and by far best option, preserves everybody's rights. Looking directly at the woman, Julie could say, "I really appreciate your concern about my having a good time. It's nice when someone takes time to show interest. But truly I kind of feel left out. See, I wish you'd talk to me directly. Please don't misinterpret what I'm saying. I do appreciate your concern, but I'd be even more grateful if you'd talk to me not about me. OK?"

The assertive way expresses feelings without alienating parties. Done eye-to-eye, respectfully, honestly, friendly, competently, considerately, and conversationally, it uses lots of " I " statements (your feelings) and minimizes "you" ones (accusations).

If you're going to try assertiveness, practice it first. Initially, practice alone by thinking about what to say and rehearsing what you decide to say. Then, practice with a friend where your partner plays the person you want to confront while you be you, and lastly, to brighten an already illuminating experience, switch roles.

Could other questions and challenges have been applied here to dispute disability assumption 1 ? Yes. It's up to you to decide what to use and when.

When trying the algorithm, don't be surprised if it takes days or weeks to complete its questions and challenges, and realize that it may take even longer for them to have their intended effects. Relatedly, you

31

may find that disability assumptions other than the one you're focused on are also depressing you. Most important, as said, think of successfully changing any one of them as a beginning, as gaining a foothold on the path towards thinking better and feeling better. Significant change takes time.

STEP 7 REAPPRAISE

Devise a fairer, more helpful way of looking at whatever triggered — incidents, comments, recollections, etc. — the nasty assumption identified. Compare your thinking now with your thinking then. Look at what you said in step three. What would you say now? You may have to think about that for a few days or weeks first.

Four days later, Julie writes, "After hearing the woman refer to me in the third person as if I was too decrepit to comprehend things, I thought of myself as looking feeble in the wheelchair, appearing as if I'd lost it, and as not being worth her time and attention like I would be if I appeared normal. All this made me angry and sad the same time. What's becoming clearer now is that "I" not "she" made me feel angry and sad. I know there are those out there who kill with kindness. They mean well, but they hurt just the same. That this woman wouldn't face me is her problem and in no way means I'm less worthy than Jacki or anyone else. If I am, it's for reasons other than my disabilities. So, instead of assuming that my disabilities diminish my worth, and there's nothing I can do about it, I'll assume that some people might treat me differently because I'm disabled, and sometimes I'll like it, and sometimes I won't, and sometimes I won't care either way. When I don't like it, I can do something about it, if I choose to. But no matter what happens, my worth as a person has nothing to do with my disability."

STEP 8 CONSIDER AGAIN THE MISERY-GENERATING ASSUMPTION IDENTIFIED AND RE-RATE HOW MUCH YOU AGREE THAT IT IS TRUE

What do you now say after having questioned and challenged the assumption and reappraised the events triggering it? Apply the scale used in step 4, and compare your responses then with those now.

To what extent do you still believe that your disability diminishes your worth and there's nothing you can do about it.

Possible ratings:

0. Not at all

1. Somewhat

2. Moderately

3. A Lot

Julie's previous rating: #3 A Lot

Julie's current rating: #1 Somewhat

STEP 9. RE-RATE THE STRENGTH OF THE EMOTIONS YOU NAMED PREVIOUSLY

As in step 2, rate from 1 to 100 the degree you feel each emotion. Compare your ratings now with those made before and note the difference, if any.

Julie's previous rating: despair (70), anger (60)

Julie's current rating: despair (20), anger (50)

Julie says, "I still feel about as angry as I did in the beginning , though I think with a little time and thought that might lessen. However, that woman was insensitive and insensitivity has always riled me and will continue to rile me. But what bothers me more than all this is my almost daily despair. When things happen to worsen it, such as what happened with the mall lady, it's comforting knowing I can do things, if I choose to. IF I CHOOSE TO, meaning it's up to me, meaning I'm not a victim. The despair that I felt over this particular incident has dropped appreciably (from 70 to 20). It will probably drop even further, if I ever do get the opportunity to be and choose to be assertive with someone like that. I'm beginning to really see that my disability has nothing to do with my worth. Seeing that and not letting myself think otherwise helps me feel I can be more in charge of what happens to me."

MS has slammed and severely shocked Julie, as it does to so many. But she has not been destroyed. Julie has made a meaningful start in improving her mood and attitude towards her disability that could if continued strengthen her resolve enough for her to eventually resume her advertising career. She understands better how her assumptions affect her moods and is comforted and empowered by knowing what to do to help herself feel better. Julie has acquired skills that with practice will help her deal with other dysfunctional assumptions that may be holding her back.

Keep At It

Sadly, there are those out there who now and probably always will ignore wheelchair- and walker-users. Never assume if they ignore you it reflects your worth. But if somewhere in your mind you do harbor that depressing misinterpretation, question and challenge it with either the methods just shown or those soon to be shown. And remember that modifying a self-denigrating assumption takes patience, time, repetition and self-scrutiny. A little nerve doesn't hurt, either.

All this became clear to me several years ago when I first started with a walker. At that time I worried that my students (college kids can be an unforgiving bunch) would think me less competent than I should be, less than the able profs. anyway, so I hid the walker in my car's trunk, using the contraption only when with friends and family. Don't know why I connected disability with diminished competence, but I did, many do. I guess I just echoed the idiocy. In any event, I did know that if I touched walls and clutched corners, I could get to and from class without falling, but also knew that the effort exacted a heavy toll: by day's-end I was overcooked spaghetti.

Something had to be done. So, ever the psychologist, I questioned, and challenged this variant of the disability diminishes worth assumption:

"If I show I'm disabled — use the walker — others will think me less competent than I should be and that's something I cannot bear, so no matter what, don't let anyone see me use the walker."

Overcoming Disabilities despair

I argued for the pluses of rejecting this assumption, such as having an easier life and saving energy, and I eventually made an assertive challenge to it and to my presumption it was unchangeable, a challenge that lifted my confidence, actually made it soar. I push-rolled into class one day and, guess what, didn't have a melt-down. If some thought my disability made me less competent, they didn't hold that view for long, at least didn't show it. In minutes, the roar of silent stares ended and a repairing, enabling, relaxing existence began for me. But I had to repeat and repeat and repeat before I really could think differently.

So probably will you. It might take six or seven or more confronts before you beat back a nasty assumption and feel better. And even then something might occur later to revive it temporarily causing a setback, a lapse. Fight the assumption again. Question and challenge it. Prevent the lapse from becoming a relapse, an abiding return to self-defeat.

You will be happier if you defeat the misery-generating disability assumptions trying to defeat you. The next chapter questions and challenges another one of them.

Overcoming Disabilities despair

CHAPTER 4 Disability Assumption 2: Disability Ends Happiness

David Perry, a 33-year-old computer analyst, left his office at exactly 5 PM on Friday 2 years, four months, and 18 days ago. He headed home along Keston. It was just getting dark. He didn't mind driving when it was dark, but driving just before dark bothered him. "It's harder to see at the time of day," he'd often tell Paula, his wife of three years. "I'm always worried that someone will smash me." Needless to say, five o'clock departures made David apprehensive. But not today. He was so eager to get home and join Paula for a special anniversary dinner and so ready to get started on the upcoming sports-filled three day weekend, which included his running a marathon, that he pushed his driving-anxiety out of his consciousness. He also forgot to buckle up.

Reaching Keston and McGillivray, traffic moving fast, the usually long light still green, David forcibly pressed pedal to metal. That's the last thing about being in his car he remembered. His next memory was screaming sirens, paramedics, speeding to the hospital, and choking fear. A drunk behind the wheel of a half ton truck had broadsided him, changing David's life forever.

David sustained injures to his spinal cord below the first thoracic spinal nerve, more specifically, at the fifth thoracic vertebrae (T5). The injury was complete, leaving him with full mobility of head, neck, and shoulders, arms, and hands, but total paralysis of legs and lower body.

In one horrible moment, David had joined the ranks of thousands with spinal cord injuries — about 8000 new cases in the United States alone every year, mostly in men under 30 and mostly from motor vehicle accidents but sometimes from mishaps as disparate as sports injuries, falls, and vicious attacks. There are many possibilities.

Regardless of how it happens, though, what eventually results depends where on the cord the spinal cord injury (SCI) is located and whether that injury is complete, like David's, or partial. The spinal cord comprises nerves entering it from the cervical, thoracic, lumbar, and sacral regions and serves as the body's communication cable. It runs from the brain down the back; bony vertebrae protect it. Basically, spinal cord injuries disrupt the brain's ability to communicate back and forth through nerves with the muscles. When the nerves injured are those entering the spinal cord in the cervical region, indicates Dr. Segun T. Dawodu, tetraplegia also called quadriplegia, paralysis of the arms and legs, results. When it's those entering the spinal cord in the thoracic and lower regions, paraplegia, paralysis of the legs, results.

The latter happened to David. His T5 damage left him a paraplegic. After months of rehabilitation, he now uses a manual wheelchair, allowing him to preserve his upper body strength, and drives a handicap adapted minivan with a lowered floor, remote control ramp for wheelchair entry, and hand controls for driving.

Grateful to have been able to return to his computer analyst job so soon after the accident, David is nonetheless sad much of the time, assuming as he does that his disabilities have quashed his chances to be happy, and that there's nothing he can do about it. "I want things the way they used to be. I want me back"; he often dreams he's once more the marathoner—fast, strong, indefatigable. The dark cloud of disabilities despair hovers over David.

Do you believe, as does David, that disability ends happiness? If you do, perhaps without realizing it you've convinced yourself that because you can't do everything you used to that was challenging and enjoyable, you can't do much of anything new that's challenging and enjoyable. Perhaps for you like for some men and women needing canes, walkers, or wheelchairs, it's all or it's nothing.

If so, I hope this chapter encourages you to start thinking differently. It will show you, through David's efforts, how to start disputing disability assumption 2 and enable yourself to find sources of pleasure and mastery that will lift your spirits.

STEP 1 DESCRIBE WHAT HAPPENED THAT UPSET YOU

Something upset you. Write down what. Possibly nothing specific you can name took place other than just thinking of things — daydreams, recollections, worries about what's to come — and your depressed mood seems to worsen or harden; detail your thoughts.

David writes, "As usual, was listening to Alan Q. on morning radio while having breakfast before work. Was feeling a bit down but not that far down until he announced that Grandview would soon be hosting a rodeo on the weekend that everyone should get tickets for early. He painted an intriguing picture of the horses, Cowboys, and bleachers. Rodeos have never been my thing, but knowing that I couldn't go even if I wanted to go because I couldn't sit in the bleachers or even get up there brought my limitations to mind, not that they're very far from it at anytime. But sometimes I don't think about them, especially when I'm doing something I enjoy like having breakfast. My disability's always there, but today after listening to Alan Q. it hit me in the face. Couldn't stop thinking about how my SCI is robbing me."

STEP 2 NAME AND RATE YOUR NEGATIVE FEELINGS

Write down your feelings — name them — and rate how strongly from 1 (hardly at all) to 100 (extremely) you feel them.

After listening to the radio, David states and rates his one main feeling as follows: despair (90)

STEP 3. IDENTIFY EACH MISERY-GENERATING ASSUMPTION TRIGGERED

Ask yourself why you feel the way you feel. To answer, try to recover the thoughts you had when the situation that upset you happened — replay your inner voice. From those thoughts search for each misery- making assumption triggered. Do each assumption separately.

David's Disabling Thoughts:

David writes, "Never used to think about whether or not I could do something — used to be quite active — but now there's denial, I mean I'm denied things others take for granted (thought 1). To me that means my shrinking world is darkening, blackening, which means pleasure is going, going, gone; no more opportunity to enjoy life (thought 2)."

Possible Disability Assumptions:

1) If I'm disabled, my worth is diminished, and there's nothing I can do about it

2) If I'm disabled, I can never be happy again, and there's nothing I can do about it

3) If I'm disabled, I look ugly, and there's nothing I can do about it

4) If I'm disabled, I'm helpless, and there's nothing I can do about it

5) If I'm disabled, I have no hope for the future, and there's nothing I can do about it

Disability Assumption Identified:

David picks, "If I'm disabled, I can never be happy again, and there's nothing I can do about it, as the closest disability assumption."

STEP 4. RATE HOW MUCH YOU AGREE THAT THE ASSUMPTION IDENTIFIED IS TRUE

For each assumption triggered, rate to what extent you agree that it is true using the scale that follows:

0. Not at all

1. Somewhat

2. Moderately

3. A Lot

David's rating: #3. A Lot *

Overcoming Disabilities despair

STEP 5. DISPUTE BY QUESTIONING THE ASSUMPTION IDENTIFIED

Dispute the assumption by questioning its value, logic, evidence or accuracy, or all these qualities.

Possible Questions to Ask:

6) What Are The Pluses of Accepting And Those of Rejecting The Assumption?
7) Would I Say it to Someone Else?
8) How Do I Figure?
9) Am I Thinking Rigidly?
10) Am I Labeling?
11) What Are The Exceptions (Search for Exceptions)?
12) Am I Fortune-telling?
13) Am I Catastrophizing?
14) Am I Letting My Feelings Be My Reality?
15) What Would a High-priced Lawyer Say?

Actual Questions Asked:

Question #10: What Would a High-priced Lawyer Say?

Sometimes it is difficult to argue on your own behalf against a misery-generating assumption because it strikes an especially hard to dispute chord within you. Before giving up, try stepping outside yourself to gain perspective. Imagine you are a lawyer in a courtroom. Cross-examine the believer of the assumption (yourself) about what it proclaims as truth. The lawyer's goal is to inject reasonable doubt into the assumption's credibility. Childish, you say? I think not. Try the exercise, you'll be surprised.

Pretend you're a lawyer given the task of arguing with yourself against assuming disability ends happiness. The assumption says disability causes lasting unhappiness and that nothing can be done to make things better. Relatedly, it suggests that disabilities must vanish or diminish before there's happiness. Argue — in writing — with

41

Overcoming Disabilities despair

yourself against the three propositions inherent in this assumption:

A. Your disability has to cause you lasting unhappiness

B. Because of your disability, you can do nothing to make yourself happy.

C. Unless your disability vanishes or diminishes significantly, you can never be happy again

Disputing: Disability must cause lasting unhappiness.

Lawyer: "Do you believe that because you are a paraplegic you can never be happy again — experience the joy that comes from doing fun things and achieving?"

David: "Yes, it seems that I do."

Lawyer: "Is it at least possible to be paralyzed as you are and not be unhappy?"

David: "It's possible."

Lawyer: "Okay, then is it possible that there are some individuals who are paraplegic who still find happiness much of the time?"

David: "I don't know every paraplegic, so I can't say for sure. But I guess it's possible."

Lawyer: "If it is possible for others, why isn't it possible for you?"

David: "I don't know, it just isn't. I love sports."

Lawyer: "Are you saying there's nobody as disabled as you who likes sports? Is there something else that makes you different from others whose legs are paralyzed, but who find happiness?"

David: "All I know is I certainly can't do the things I used to do, and there's nothing new for me out there."

Reasonable doubt has been established to the claim that paraplegia must lead to lasting unhappiness, for likely there are those who are paraplegic who find ways to be happy.

Disputing: I can do nothing to make myself happy

Overcoming Disabilities despair

Lawyer: "Is there absolutely nothing enjoyable you can do now that you used to do?"

David: "Well, I used to love to play basketball and run marathons. If your legs are paralyzed, your marathon days are over for sure."

Lawyer: "Maybe so, in the traditional way, but aren't there many individuals who enjoy sports in wheelchairs?"

David: "Yes of course, but for me that would be way too hard."

Lawyer: "Okay, but even if that's too strenuous for you, aren't there many fun activities, like going to dinner, concerts, or plays, and achievement-activities—sources of fulfillment—like writing, taking courses, mastering chess, and much much more that you could do and might like to do?"

David: "Possibly.

Lawyer: "Do you agree that such things are enjoyed by some persons with SCI who need wheelchairs?"

David: "Definitely."

Lawyer: "Well, if you agree that there are many enjoyable and fulfilling activities that some others whose legs are paralyzed enjoy, is there any reason why you can't be one of them and derive pleasure and satisfaction from being active?"

David: "I don't know."

Lawyer: "Is it possible that there are things you haven't tried, haven't given thought to, that if done would be pleasurable or at least satisfying?"

David: "Probably."

Lawyer: "For you to conclude that the opportunities to be happy are gone, wouldn't you first have to try and fail at many opportunities for pleasure and achievement?"

David: "I guess so."

Lawyer: "Have you tried and failed at numbers of these sorts of

43

activities?"

David: "No, haven't tried."

Reasonable doubt established to the part of the assumption claiming that nothing can be done: quite likely, there are pleasurable and fulfilling activities available to try, and there have been insufficient attempts to try them.

Disputing: Only if disability vanishes or diminishes significantly is happiness possible.

Lawyer: "Why do you think you're unhappy?"

David: "Because I'm disabled."

Lawyer: "What, in your mind, is the relationship between disability and happiness?"

David: "Disability means can't do, and SCI disability like mine is forever, and can't do forever spells an end to happiness forever."

Lawyer: "Are you also saying that because your disability won't diminish—in your words it's forever—you're going to remain unhappy?"

David: "Definitely."

Lawyer: "So in your case happiness mostly or entirely has to do with disability?"

David: "Yes."

Lawyer: "Is it possible though to change your way of thinking about being disabled—your assumptions and attitudes—and by so doing improve your mood?"

David: "Perhaps."

Lawyer: "And isn't it possible that if your mood would improve, you'd look at the world differently and find more joy in living?"

David: "Maybe."

Reasonable doubt established to the implication that only if disability vanishes or diminishes significantly will happiness be possible.

Question #1: What Are The Pluses Of Accepting and Those of Rejecting The Assumption "I can never be happy again, and there's nothing I can do about it"?

Look closely at the assumption.

What does accepting it do for you?

What does rejecting it do for you?

Do the pluses of rejecting outnumber or outweigh, or both outnumber and outweigh, those of accepting?

If the pluses of rejecting are greater, likely they are, you have put into question the assumption's utility for you and by so doing siphoned a bit of its power over you.

David writes, "If I accept this assumption, I won't have to leave my comfortable home when I'm not at work and be a part of anything. Right now, with my fatigue, that's a real plus. Also, if I accept this assumption, I won't have to spend money doing things; my budget is tight. As well, I won't have to go out and be noticed, pitied — things I hate.

But if I reject this assumption, I have given myself that important nudge to try to recapture some of what I used to have and hold onto what I still have and learn new things. By trying, I will help myself overcome this feeling of being robbed. I can be like some other paraplegics who find many opportunities for experiencing pleasure and feelings of mastery. The really significant plus of rejecting this assumption is that Paula and I can do more together. Clearly there are pluses on both sides. But those of accepting the assumption take me nowhere, those of rejecting it take me to a better place."

Question #2: Would I Say it to Someone Else?

Harder on yourself than on others? If you are, ask why the double standard, one for you and one for the rest of us, and the unfairness of

45

what you're doing cries out. David writes, "I seem to be telling myself that it's game over, something I wouldn't say to a friend with my disabilities about his or her chances for happiness. June's brother, Tom, has a spinal cord injury almost like mine, and I certainly wouldn't tell him you're a paraplegic therefore you'd better stay home and watch daytime TV or listen to radio tapes—get used to that. Find a lot of good books because you're finished. Don't even attempt anything new.

Saying that would be pretty damning, cruel, and needless. So why do I tell myself things like that? Instead, I should tell Tom that I know he feels rough, but to give-in is to give-up. I also would tell him that I'm sure there are things he can't do and wants to do, but I'm betting there are things he doesn't do that he could do, things that would give him pleasure and power. SCI is not the end of you. It can be a beginning of new ways of self understanding and achievement.

I have got to start talking to me as good as I would talk to Tom."

STEP 6 DISPUTE BY CHALLENGING THE ASSUMPTION IDENTIFIED

Dispute by challenging behaviorally the part that says, "and there's nothing I can do about it."

Possible Challenges to Make:

1) Challenge by Assertiveness

2) Challenge by Activation

3) Challenge by Problem-solving

4) Challenge by Contracting

5) Challenge by Relaxation

6) Challenge by Exposure

Actual Challenges Made:

Challenge #2: The Activation Challenge

Sadness breeds sadness. It does so when, to the sad individual, doing nothing becomes more attractive than doing something. By engineering experiences of pleasure and mastery, activation replaces doing little or nothing and feeling lousy with doing more and feeling better. Here's how to activate:

Step #1 Take a baseline. How active are you? Learn where you are so you can set your sights on where to go.

For one week, list what you do activity-by-activity during five or six three-hour intervals throughout the day and evening; just note sleeping—4, 6, 8 hours, whatever.

Rate how pleasurable each activity you did was.

Let 0=no pleasure, 5=moderately pleasurable, 10=the most pleasure you can think of. So, your rating of how pleasurable doing a certain something was will be somewhere between 0 & 10.

Place this number immediately after the activity recorded.

Likewise, rate how much of a mastery feeling (sense of achievement, competency, effectiveness, independence) doing it gave you.

Use the same sort of zero to ten system where 0=no mastery, 5=a moderate amount, 10=the most you can imagine.

Place this number after the pleasure rating (e.g.,breakfasting, 3/0).

Before listing all his activities on a baseline form, David writes, "Got up early, even though it's Saturday. After dressing, went down and had breakfast. I enjoyed breakfast, so I gave it a 6 for pleasure, but of course got no sense of mastery from it, so gave it a 0 for mastery [6/0]. The most pleasure I had today was when Jen came home bubbling and excitedly said (she could hardly get the words out) she scored a soccer goal at morning practice. She's my treasure, so I rated the pleasure I got from her as 9. I'm really proud of her."

BASELINE ACTIVITIES Day Sat Date Mar 20
7am to 10am • breakfast 6/0 • watched 2 ½ hours of TV sports (2/0
After 10am to 1pm • 3 hrs. of football on TV 4/0
After 1pm to 4pm • lunch 4/0 • read novel 3/2
After 4pm to 7pm • Jen and I talked about her soccer practice 9/3 • listened to music CD's 5/1 • Dinner 4/0
After 7pm to 10pm • 3 hrs.TV 4/0 • Bed (7 hrs.)

After reviewing his baseline record, David notes, "One thing clear to me is that there is not a lot of pleasure or mastery in my life right now. Maybe that will change if I build some experiences that I can enjoy and feel good about. I don't get a lot of exercise, and that bothers me. I can certainly exercise more.

Step #2: Plan more activity. One source of activities is your baseline record. Look it over and devise a livable, reasonable increase in daily activities; have the increase cover two weeks. When activating, look for behaviors—lifters—that give you a sense of mastery (achievement, effectiveness, independence, triumph) or pleasure, or both mastery and pleasure.

Fill your life with lifters. Fun-stuff, such as going to movies, dining well, attending a concert, the list goes on, certainly qualify as lifters. But lifters like these may not provide much in the way of mastery, unless doing them is for you a real achievement—if depressed and unable to do more than watch TV on the weekend, getting out and doing something, anything, will be a real achievement. Seek pleasure and mastery.

Activate the lifters, but equally important, deactivate the downers—behaviors such as watching TV during the day, everyday, that temporarily relieve boredom yet won't lift mood beyond the length of the show. The escape is fleeting .When you plan, Set small goals, but gradually do more and more.

For each activity you plan, predict how much pleasure you expect from doing it (e.g., 0=no pleasure, 5=moderately pleasurable, 10=the most pleasure you can think of).

Predict as well, how much mastery you anticipate (e.g.,0=no mastery, 5=a moderate amount, 10= the most you can imagine).

Place both numbers (e.g., exercising 20 minutes,3/2) immediately after the planned activity in the planned column of your data-keeping form.

Step #3: Do the activities planned. As soon as convenient after completing a planned activity, record that you've done it in the "Completed" column. Use the previously described pleasure and mastery rating system to say how much of each you actually experienced (e.g., exercising 20 minutes, 4/5). For sleeping and other activities that take a long time or for those you've planned but haven't completed, just note the particulars on the form. David's activity form follows:

Overcoming Disabilities despair

ACTIVITIES PLANNED AND COMPLETED

Day: Sat Date March 27

Planned	Completed
7-10am	**7-10am**
1 hr. information radio 2/1	1 hr. information radio 2/2
Call Tom & ask about local wheelchair marathons 5/2	Call Tom & learned about wheelchair marathons nearby. telephoned marathon office 6/6
Lift dumbbells 20min 3/2	Lifted DB 20 minutes 4/5
Chk internet for wheelchair marathons 3/4	checked for wheelchair marathons 4/5
After 10am-1pm	**After 10am-1pm**
visit Art gallery with Paula 4/5	Visited Art gallery 4/5
After 1pm-4pm	**After 1pm-4pm**
tidy home office & take out garbage 1/6	cleaned home office & took out out garbage 1/6
movie with Jen at Cineplex 6/3	Jen and I had great time at movie 8/3
After 4pm-7pm	**After 4pm-7pm**
play Clue & Risk with Jen and Paula 8/3	Clue & Risk with Jen and Paula 8/7
Dinner 4/0	Dinner 4/0
After 7pm-11pm	**After 7pm-11pm**
TV 4/0	TV 3/0
make popcorn 4/4	made popcorn 4/5
Bed (7hrs.)	Bed (6 hrs.)

[Blank baseline and planned/completed forms are included at end of the book.]

At first, you might have to force yourself to activate, to slowly do more and more each day so pleasure and mastery have a chance to reward. As you do activate, be mindful of activation-stoppers---plan-killers—like fatigue. David invoked it as reason, one of a few, to accept disability assumption 2. He didn't want to activate because he was too fatigued to leave his house when not at work. Frequently, the more dispirited one is, the more tired one feels, and the less one wants to activate, but activation can energize you. Fatigue, a disabilities side effect chapter 8 will more fully address, works against its own solution.

Another plan-killer is overplanning, planning so much and feeling so overburdened that you don't want to do anything. Motivation to fulfill the plan drains away. Do your best to stay motivated. If unable to pinpoint why you may no longer have the drive to continue, try giving yourself a few bucks towards something desirable for living up to the plan. Some folks would say that such self-reward is just bribing yourself, but if a few dollars helps keep you activated, take the bribe. We'll soon discuss a convenient system of self-reward, actually a disability assumption challenge, called behavioral contracting.

Yet another plan-killer, a roadblock to activating, is fear. Suppose, you have planned an outing with friends at a downtown museum which you think is a six in pleasure and a three in mastery (6/3); friends tell you the place is handicap accessible. Relying upon a walker, you worry, I'll fall down and then what, so you decide not to go. But what's the likelihood of falling down? How often does that really happen to you? Falling down is a possibility not an inevitability. And even if it happens, will it so devastate you that recovery is impossible? Will there be no one to help? Sometimes you can reason away a fear that's blocking your progress.

But many times you can't. Many fears are stubborn and require a direct attack through exposure, a behavioral tool chapter 9 will exemplify.

STEP 7. REAPPRAISE

Devise a fairer, more helpful way of looking at whatever triggered— incidents, comments, recollections, etc.—the nasty assumption identified. Compare your thinking now with your thinking then. Look at what you said in step three. What would you say now? You may have to think about that for a few days or weeks first.

David reappraises his thinking after disputing assumption 2 and writes, "I wouldn't have fun at a rodeo, even if I could get there and sit there. Never liked things like that anyway. But what bugs me is the CAN'T go. True, things have changed . But just because I can't do some things, doesn't mean I can't do all things. Won't give-up looking. Won't give-up on me. My chances to enjoy life are not over. I'll assume that I can still feel pleasure and mastery if I search for and create the right opportunities for them. I know it's tougher now, but it's still up to me."

STEP 8. CONSIDER AGAIN THE MISERY-GENERATING ASSUMPTION IDENTIFIED AND RE-RATE HOW MUCH YOU AGREE THAT IT IS TRUE

What do you now say after having questioned and challenged the assumption and reappraised the events triggering it? Apply the scale used in step 4, and compare your responses then with those now.

To what extent do you still believe that disability ends happiness, and there's nothing you can do about it.

Possible ratings:

0. Not at all

1. Somewhat

2. Moderately

3. A Lot

David's previous rating: #3 A Lot

David's current rating: #1 Somewhat

STEP 9. RE-RATE THE STRENGTH OF THE EMOTIONS YOU NAMED PREVIOUSLY

As in step 2, rate from 1 to 100 the degree you feel each emotion. Compare your ratings now with those made before and note the difference, if any.

Overcoming Disabilities despair

David's previous rating: despair (90)

David's current rating: despair (20)

David writes, "That's a 70 point drop, and to me significant; it's the difference between living with overwhelming despair or manageable despair. I don't for a minute delude myself into believing I'll ever be totally okay about things I cannot do, even if I really would not be first in line to do them — still have and probably always will have the if-others-can-why-can't-I feeling. But I have to teach myself over and over again that "can't do" on some things is not "can't do" on all things — that in this world there's much for me to enjoy and be proud of.

I won't let my non-functioning legs silence my functioning brain."

David has been dealt a bad hand, and understandably he wishes it were not so.

But if he surrenders to his unhappiness, he's guaranteed sadness and despair for the rest of his days. What he has done by disputing disability assumption 2 is what Julie did in the previous chapter with disability assumption 1: make a significant start towards overcoming recurrent disabilities despair. Neither can be assured of continuous uninterrupted progress. There will be pitfalls and setbacks. Yet by proving to themselves they can relinquish the victim's mentality of there's nothing I can do about it for the survivor's mentality of doing something about it, Julie and David have become a little stronger, a little more empowered, a little more resilient. Each has taken a major step, albeit an initial step, towards greater well-being.

And so can you. Dispute the assumptions putting you down and holding you back. Question and challenge them. Three questions and one challenge have been used here, there are others, as chapters to come illustrate.

Overcoming Disabilities despair

CHAPTER 5 Disability Assumption 3: Disability Means Ugly

Alexandria Koulack-Wilson, Ally for short, has three strikes against her, and she's not yet even 40 years old . She feels the effects of disability assumption 3 most acutely because of the third strike, but each strike has contributed to her negative outlook because each strike, like dominoes in a line, has set the stage for the next.

Strike 1

When Ally was six years old in an all girl first-grade, the teacher told her and the other children that Ally should be that year's class Santa because, in teachers words, "Ally has more meat on her bones." Liking the attention but somewhat confused, Ally didn't know if being the class Santa Claus was an honor or a slight. Santa Clauses were fat, and Ally was definitely the heaviest girl in class. She remained the heaviest or almost the heaviest of her classmates throughout grammar school and high school. In college, as well, she was overweight. On the day she married Peter, three weeks before her 30th birthday, Ally weighed 160 pounds and stood 5'1". Her body mass index (BMI), computed by multiplying her weight in pounds by 703 and dividing the result by her height in inches squared, was 30.2.

[BMI = (pounds x 703)/ height 2 (inches)].

160 lb x 703 = 112480/ (3721)

BMI = 30.2

That's a high BMI, and a high BMI correlates with a panoply of health problems, including but not limited to heart disease, asthma, some types of cancer, and type II diabetes. Health professionals say BMIs under 25 are normal, 25 to 29.9 overweight, 30 to 39.9 obese and 40 or greater extremely obese. So, Ally's first strike was obesity, and it set the stage for the second strike.

Strike 2

One day, just after her 34th birthday, Ally visited her doctor for a checkup. To almost anyone who'd ask, Ally would say she was feeling fine, but there were minor, to her anyway minor, things happening. She felt frequent urges to urinate and was more tired than ever before. Though these problems were not incapacitating, they bothered Ally, so she reported them. The doctor was somewhat alarmed upon hearing about them, for such symptoms experienced by someone Ally's weight suggested a metabolic problem, namely, type II diabetes—non-insulin-dependent diabetes mellitus (NIDDM). Even though Ally had no family history of diabetes, her obesity was a significant risk factor for it.

Medical tests indeed confirmed she was a type II diabetic. The glucose her body produced from the foods she ate was not leaving her bloodstream as it should to supply vital muscle, fat, and liver cells with energy; glucose is fuel, energy, for these cells, and it wasn't reaching them. Her body was not properly responding to the insulin her pancreas made; insulin is a hormone needed for the glucose to get to the cells. This unresponsiveness resulted in higher than desirable blood glucose levels, a clear sign of diabetes.

Ally's form of diabetes, type II, is the most common— about 90% of diabetics have it in contrast to type I, insulin-dependent diabetes mellitus (IDDM). Those with type I diabetes are not obese but have deficient supplies of insulin. With type I diabetes, be it in children or adults, the pancreas does not make any or enough insulin. In contrast, Ally's body produced enough insulin, but for some reason wouldn't allow it to do its job. Strike two on Ally, brought on by her obesity, was type II diabetes, and it set the stage for the third strike.

Strike 3

"Oh Lord, what's happening, pins and needles in my leg, left side of my face drooping, feel like throwing up, so dizzy." Ally was home, just getting ready to go to work when all this started. Calling Peter on his cell, panic in her voice, she begged for help. Her slurred speech scared him. So, while talking to Ally on his cell, trying to calm her, he dialed 911 on his desk phone. Paramedics reached Ally in minutes; she and Peter were still talking when they arrived .

Ally was having an ischemic stroke from a clot blocking the flow of oxygen to her brain. Rapid treatment by the hospital's stroke trauma unit prevented her from dying, but not from sustaining damage to her brain's right hemisphere, resulting in, among other challenges, left leg immobility with a pronounced left foot drop. Strike three on Ally, made decidedly more inevitable by her type II diabetes, was a stroke.

After much rehabilitation, she was able to return to work and recover nearly all of her ability to speak. However, she needed an orthotic device, leg brace, which she could wear under her clothes and a cane to walk. The highly visible cane made her extremely uncomfortable when among coworkers because she perceived their looks to be stares of discomfort and pity. So, she requested a private space to work where she would have few contacts with others. As well, she avoided most meetings and group activities, lunched alone, stopped going to the gym, and became what she later would term "a junk-food junkie." Her main relief from misperceived public scrutiny was hiding out at home when she could and eating high calorie junk foods. The solitude and eating comforted her.

Ally was assuming that disability means ugly. In order to dispute that assumption, or at least begin to dispute it, she worked through the nine step algorithm after experiencing the following incident:

STEP 1 DESCRIBE WHAT HAPPENED THAT UPSET YOU

Something upset you. Write down what. Possibly nothing specific you can name took place other than just thinking of things — daydreams, recollections, worries about what's to come — and your depressed mood seems with worsen or harden; detail your thoughts.

Ally writes, "Putting a cane in my hand is putting a sign on me that says, 'look here I am, watch me walk', as if a heavy lady approaching 40 with a bum left leg really needed that. Made up my mind in high school that I can't compete with all the large-breasted bean poles. Can't remember ever being thin or normal and not wishing I were — tried 100 diets, nothing works, but since my stroke, I've come to really loath my body. I've gained 35 pounds. That's not good for my health, I know. Scares my doctor, could have another stroke, but I just feel what's the use. Can't do anything about it, can't do anything about me, just don't have the drive to do all that. Don't think Peter is turned on by me anymore. He says he still is.

What brought all this stuff to me more vividly and just deepened the black hole I've been in ever since I began with a cane is really stupid. It was just that blond kid this morning at the market. I asked Peter to go shopping but he couldn't, so I had to, even if really didn't want to. The blond boy couldn't have been more than six years-old. When he saw me hobbling, his eyes grew wide. He stared at me as if I'd just jumped out at him from one of his scary books. The way he looked at me really got to me. His mom told him not to stare, but ignoring her he shouted, 'Who's she? Why's she walk like that?' Embarrassing. His words still sting."

STEP 2 NAME AND RATE YOUR NEGATIVE FEELINGS

Write down your feelings - name them - and rate how strongly from 1 (hardly at all) to 100 (extremely) you feel them.

After the episode at the market, Ally states and rates her feelings as follows: despair (90), ugly (100), futility (90)

STEP 3 IDENTIFY EACH MISERY-GENERATING ASSUMPTION TRIGGERED

Ask yourself why you feel the way you feel. To answer, try to recover the thoughts you had when the situation that upset you happened — replay your inner voice. From those thoughts search for each misery-making assumption triggered. Do each assumption separately.

Ally's Disabling Thoughts:

Ally writes, "My thought was I look weird to him and probably to everyone else, too."

Possible Disability Assumptions:

1) If I'm disabled, my worth is diminished, and there's nothing I can do about it

2) If I'm disabled, I can never be happy again, and

Overcoming Disabilities despair

there's nothing I can do about it

3) If I'm disabled, I look ugly, and there's nothing I can do about it

4) If I'm disabled, I'm helpless, and there's nothing I can do about it

5) If I'm disabled, I have no hope for the future, and there's nothing I can do about it

Disability Assumption Identified:

Ally says, "There's no doubt in my mind what assumption is responsible for that way of thinking: I look ugly."

STEP 4. RATE HOW MUCH YOU AGREE THAT THE ASSUMPTION IDENTIFIED IS TRUE

For each assumption triggered, rate to what extent you agree that it is true using the following scale:

0. Not at all

1. Somewhat

2. Moderately

3. A Lot

Ally's rating: A Lot

STEP 5. DISPUTE BY QUESTIONING THE ASSUMPTION IDENTIFIED

Dispute the assumption by questioning its value, logic, fairness, evidence, or accuracy, or all these qualities.

Possible Questions To Ask:

1) What Are The Pluses of Accepting And Those of Rejecting The Assumption?

2) Would I Say it to Someone Else?

3) How Do I Figure?

4) Am I Thinking Rigidly?

5) Am I Labeling?

6) What Are The Exceptions (Search for Exceptions)?

7) Am I Fortune-telling?

8) Am I Catastrophizing?

9) Am I Letting My Feelings Be My Reality?

10) What Would a High-priced Lawyer Say?

Actual Questions Asked:

Question #4: Am I Thinking Rigidly?

Rigid thinking is black and white thinking, all or nothing thinking, success or failure thinking; it overlooks the freeing in-betweens, the shades of gray so necessary to accurate appraisal. Cognitive-behavior therapists observe that categorical thinking (you're good or bad, right or wrong, helpless or helpful) promotes inflexibility and stifles thinking both of which can lead to self-deprecation and despair.

Ally writes,: "Guess I'm thinking in categories of either/or — either I look good or I look ugly, and that way of thinking gets me blue. Walking with a cane certainly doesn't make me appealing but it doesn't make me ugly, either. I'm not now nor have I ever been movie star material, but that doesn't mean I'm a beauty shop reject, bleeding from open sores; I walk with a cane."

Question #9: Am I Letting My Feelings Be My Reality?

It's logical for reality to influence, even define feelings. How you live and what befalls you will greatly affect your emotions. But it's illogical to let feelings define reality — to let how you feel represent what in fact is. Yet that is what numbers of depressed individuals do, a misery-generating style of thinking that, as said, many cognitive behavior- therapists call emotional reasoning.

Ally writes, "Sometimes I see my reflection and really do feel ugly. That's just the way I feel. But what proof do I have that that's really the way things are, that I really am that way? I do get looks from gals at work and guys, too, even though I try to stay in my little cubbyhole. Their expressions are just as likely, more likely, to be neutral or compassionate. No one tells me or gives me the impression they think

I'm ugly, except that kid, and I think I just surprised him as much as anything else. Because I feel a certain way when I see myself does not mean that others feel that way when they see me. My feelings are not necessarily my reality."

Question #2: Would I Say It to Someone Else?

Harder on yourself than on others? If you are, ask why the double standard, one for you and one for the rest of us, and the unfairness of what you're doing cries-out.

Ally writes, "Yes clearly I 'm harder on myself than I'd be on someone else as disabled as me. I basically tell myself that the way I get about makes me ugly — even repulsive to some; hobbling with a cane is a real turnoff. But I see other disabled people, and never would I tell any of them that. Would not, could not. If they're ugly, it' s not due to the way they get around. Why then do I denigrate myself that way?"

STEP 6 DISPUTE BY CHALLENGING THE ASSUMPTION IDENTIFIED

Dispute the assumption by challenging behaviorally the part that says, "and there's nothing I can do about it." Make a challenge to that part, refute or cast reasonable doubt on it, by doing something constructive.

Possible Challenges to Make:

1) Challenge by Assertiveness

2) Challenge by Activation

3) Challenge by Problem-solving

4) Challenge by Contracting

5) Challenge by Relaxation

6) Challenge by Exposure

Actual Challenges Made:

Challenge # 4: The Contracting Challenge

Promises, promises. We make them, we break them. How many

Overcoming Disabilities despair

New Year's Eve resolutions have you kept? By itself, resolving to do something is a poor way of trying to get it done — no specifics, too few details. Much better is contracting. The contract, best when written, articulates the promises to be kept, the rewards for keeping them, and the consequences for not doing so. Nothing is vague. Contracts are agreements. You agree to do something for something.

Contracting can help you activate, be assertive, and to excel, that is, be the best that you can be intellectually, socially, and physically. Contracting can help challenge the assumption that disability makes you forever ugly, forever unattractive, forever unimprovable. In so doing, contracting impugns the "it's- no-use-why-bother" attitude, a despair-making and motivation-draining sense of futility that inhibits self-care and self-improvement.

Ally writes, "I know I'll never walk much better than I do, the hobbling and the wobbling isn't pretty. But that neither means I'm ugly nor unable to look better. One thing I can do that will help me boost my health and self-confidence is to lose 10 pounds — a good first step. I hate how my clothes fit now more than ever since gaining 35 pounds. This time, though, I'll do things right — no crazy starving myself diets, no live-or-die-50-pounds-off plan, where I die. This time things will be different."

Instead of just resolving to get off the drastic dieting treadmill, contract to do it. To understand what to put into the contract, monitor for a week what you eat and how much exercise you do. Let's say you consume 3000 calories daily, exercise occasionally, and snack frequently — candy kisses when near a prominently displayed TV-room dish and potato-chips when watching TV. Using this information, give yourself points backed-up by funds to buy new clothes for snacking better, moving more, and the like.

Here's a weight-management contract for losing 10 pounds. It lists behaviors that promote losing weight — do's — and behaviors to avoid — don'ts; the don'ts promote gaining weight or staying the same or behaving unhealthily. The contract also lists consequences: points and new clothes. Basically, Ally will earn points for doing what she promises; these earnings can be cashed in for new clothes. And Ally will lose points if she does something she has promised not to do,

Overcoming Disabilities despair

something unhealthy or unwholesome.

Do's, Don'ts, and Consequences:

- Losing 1-2 pounds a week gets 2pts/wk
- Losing 3 or more pounds a week forfeits 2 pts
- Consuming 1900-1950 calories/day gets 2pts/day.
- Consuming less than 1900 calories/day loses 2pts/day.
- Consuming less than 1000 calories/day loses 20pts/day.
- Snacking on potato chips but not exceeding ½ bag per week gets 3pts/wk.
- Not snacking on candy kisses gets 1pt/day.
- Not snacking, except on veggies and fruit, while watching TV, gets 3pts/day.
- Lifting light weights 20 minutes/day gets 3pts/ day.
- Walking with Peter in the evening 30 minutes/day gets 4 pts/day.

Points and what they buy. Point earnings can be cashed in any time:

25=white blouse

35=new runners

50=new boots

25=black pants

25=teal green ribbed-neck tunic

28=lined jeans

24=regular jeans

25=silk turtleneck

50=Irish wool sweater

40=lamb's wool sweater

25=rugby shirt

40=warm-up suit

20=lambs-wool scarf

20=pink sleep-shirt

30=denim front-wrap skirt

40=gray cardigan

Some tips for writing strong, health-giving weight-change contracts:

Write down each clause of the contract, spelling out the promises — the do's and the don'ts.

When spelling out the promises, say specifically what actions earn how many rewards, and what actions cost and how much.

Don't set out to lose more than 1 pound per week.

Avoid weight loss scams — potions and pills and exercise gimmicks.

Sign the contract to make a written commitment.

Say when earnings (points) may be cashed-in.

Use strong rewards.

Eat better and exercise more. Here are a few suggestions to help you do that:

Remove ready-to-eat snacks from your home. Give those who object to that their own snacks-containers.

- Remove snack foods from work.
- Avoid coffee and tea until that hour of the day when they won't trigger extra eating.
- List such pleasant things as telephoning a friend, taking a bath, walking, writing a letter to replace giving into cravings.

Overcoming Disabilities despair

- Plan what to buy before you shop.
- Serve less food; ask all servers to do so.
- Store leftovers in opaque containers; better to throw leftovers out then eat them if you don't want them.
- Collect menus of favorite restaurants and decide what to eat before going to any of them.
- Keep veggies and fruits handy.
- Avoid, if possible, time-to-kill situations where you pass time by eating. If they're unavoidable, carry fruits or veggies as substitutes for candybars, and so forth.
- Pack fruits and veggies for long car trips.
- Ask waiters not to serve bread before the meal.
- Avoid gnawing hunger; it's easier to reward yourself with food when hunger torments.
- Plan your exercising—when, where, with whom.

List alternative exercises (and times and places) for bad weather days and times your child, spouse, or friend forces you to abandon activity plans.

- Vary activities to avoid getting bored exercising.
- Redo the contract after a few weeks of no behavior change, but don't throw it out if you occasionally fail to keep promises.
- Say what ends the contract—a particular date or amount of weight loss.
- Not all contracts for self-improvement need be complex. Nor do all rely upon external incentives, like new clothes; signs of progress are rewarding in and of themselves.

STEP 7. REAPPRAISE

Devise a fairer, more helpful way of looking at whatever triggered— incidents, comments, recollections, etc.—the nasty assumption identified. Compare your thinking now with your thinking then. Look at what you said in step three. What would you say now? You may have to think about that for a few days or weeks first.

It didn't take Ally long to write, "I refuse to delude myself into believing the disabled-look isn't unattractive. It is unappealing. But I can't let myself feel ugly just because I don't walk normally. If I do, I close down opportunities to better myself. Also, I increase the chances of misinterpreting every lingering look from someone else as a sign I'm ugly. Perhaps I scared that child at the market, perhaps I aroused his curiosity, perhaps I reminded him of a storybook character that he feared. Whatever. His view of me is unlikely to be everyone's view."

STEP 8. CONSIDER AGAIN THE MISERY-GENERATING ASSUMPTION IDENTIFIED AND RE-RATE HOW MUCH YOU AGREE THAT IT IS TRUE

What do you now say after having questioned and challenged the assumption and reappraised the events triggering it? Apply the scale used in step 4, and compare your responses then with those now. To what extent do you still believe that disability equals ugliness, and there's nothing you can do about it.

Possible ratings:

0. Not at all

1. Somewhat

2. Moderately

3. A Lot

Ally's previous rating: #3 A Lot

Ally's current rating: #2 Moderately

STEP 9. RE-RATE THE STRENGTH OF THE EMOTIONS YOU NAMED PREVIOUSLY

As in step 2, rate from 1 to 100 the degree you feel each emotion. Compare your ratings now with those in step two and note the difference, if any.

Ally's previous ratings: despair (90), ugly (100), futility (90)

Ally's current ratings: despair (45), ugly (60), futility (20)

Ally says, "All the negative emotions are less negative now and will I hope continue to lessen. I'm sure I'll like my body more when I lose another 10 pounds or so, and I know I'll feel better and reduce the chances of another stroke if I lose more weight and keep exercising. I know who I am is not what I weigh or how I walk. I can't give up on me. I won't stop trying to improve myself in every way I can."

Ally's assumption that walking with a cane made her ugly compounded her already bad body image and intensified her feelings of despair and futility. Arguing against and effectively challenging that destructive assumption is a beginning that will lift her spirits and empower her. Continuing to argue against and challenge it will reinforce these improvements and help overcome any new crippling feelings of futility that arise, feelings that if unchecked would interfere with her becoming and staying healthier.

Ally has three strikes against her, but she's far from striking out.

Overcoming Disabilities despair

CHAPTER 6 Disability Assumption 4: Disability Means Helpless

Many individuals disabled by rheumatoid arthritis (RA) assume disability means helpless. Matthias Wilson, 50-years-old, married, two children in a nearby college and retired because of disability after almost 30 years at the phone company, does.

Like Julie Anne Jonah, the woman with MS, Matthias Wilson is his own worst enemy when it comes to what his body does without his say-so. Both Julie and Matthias have systemic autoimmune diseases. Their immune systems behave as if under attack by some foreign invader and so mistakenly attack their body's own tissues. For Julie, this undeserved aggression has resulted in her losing the precious myelin lining her nerves. For Matthias, it has resulted in his depositing inflammatory cells in the synovial fluid lubricating his joints. Julie has MS, Matthias has RA. Medical scientists don't know for sure why the immune system goes awry or why it attacks the tissues it attacks, but sometimes it just does.

All that Matthias understands about RA is that his fingers hands, wrists, and knees are painfully sore and stiff particularly in the morning but often throughout the day, and sometimes it's hard for him to grip anything. Lately, there are times when the swelling in these joints is so intense he can't stand even the slightest pressure on them. When that swollen, red and warm, the really bad days, he'll ask his wife for help getting dressed. Matthias also has three peculiar little, thankfully painless, lumps — rheumatoid nodules — on the outer side of his left elbow; not every RA sufferer gets them. As well, Matthias has a very dry mouth, a symptom of Sjögren's syndrome, which accompanies RA in some individuals; to keep his speech from slurring, he sucks on sugarless mints. The dentist attributes Matthias' cavity-increase to the Sjögren's syndrome.

Matthias believes his RA will steadily worsen despite the drug treatment he receives. Indeed, it did start out as just some muscle pain, a mild fever, and fatigue but within the last two years has noticeably worsened. So, Matthias's pessimism may be warranted, although his rheumatologist is more upbeat because experience has taught the doctor that RA is unpredictable. Some with it go steadily downhill, some fluctuate between good and bad times, and some get better and stay better. To say who will experience which course is often unclear.

Nonetheless, Matthis is convinced his life is an approaching train wreck. He's beset with feelings of helplessness and hopelessness. It's the former unpleasantness that we'll look at in this chapter and the latter in the next.

Like many do, Matthias prizes independence, strength, and self-reliance. He would be the first to tell you that in our world you better have these qualities. Can you be disabled and have them? Until recently, Matthias would firmly but despairingly maintain you can't, a pessimism causing him undeserved psychological pain. Here's how he's trying to become more realistic and optimistic.

STEP 1 DESCRIBE WHAT HAPPENED THAT UPSET YOU

Something upset you. Write down what. Possibly nothing specific you can name took place other than just thinking of things—daydreams, recollections, worries about what's to come—and your depressed mood seems to worsen or harden; detail your thoughts.

Matthias writes, "Since I left the phone company, took the disability package, my mood has been in the dumper. Wednesday evening it dropped down another notch when I read of yet another home invasion. According to the paper, three 20-year-olds, one a woman, barged into an old couple's home in broad daylight and not only robbed them of $50, but clubbed the 80-year-old man and pushed him down the stairs. Horrible. Cruel. Unnecessary. I really got mad. Those vicious miscreants, after having served only eight months for a previous home invasion, had just been paroled by government idiots. No one is safe, especially the old or the crippled. It was then, even though still madder than anything, that my ever-present despair over having RA worsened, and a naked sense of vulnerability enveloped me once again."

STEP 2. NAME AND RATE YOUR NEGATIVE FEELINGS

Write down your feelings — name them — and how strongly you feel each of them from 1 to 100 (extremely).

After reading the paper and becoming upset, Matthias states and rates his feelings as follows: vulnerability (90), fear (70), despair (80), anger (90).

STEP 3. IDENTIFY EACH MISERY-GENERATING ASSUMPTION TRIGGERED

Ask yourself why you feel the way you feel. To answer, try to recover the thoughts you had when the situation that upset you happened — replay your inner voice. From those thoughts search for each misery-making assumption triggered. Do each assumption separately.

Matthias's Disabling Thoughts:

Matthias writes, "My first thought was: with the justice system the way it is, people like me are just sheep waiting for slaughter. After a little probing I came up with: I can't watch out for me like I used to. A little more searching and I heard my father's voice saying a man has to be able to take care of himself and his family. That, I can no longer do."

Possible Disability Assumptions:

1) If I'm disabled, my worth is diminished, and there's nothing I can do about it

2) If I'm disabled, I can never be happy again, and there's nothing I can do about it

3) If I'm disabled, I look ugly, and there's nothing I can do about it

4) If I'm disabled, I'm helpless, and there's nothing I can do about it

5) If I'm disabled, I have no hope for the future, and there's nothing I can do about it

Disability Assumption Identified:

Matthias writes that to him the closest underlying assumption is: if I have disabling RA, I'm helpless, and there's nothing I can do about it

STEP 4. RATE HOW MUCH YOU AGREE THAT THE ASSUMPTION IDENTIFIED IS TRUE

For each assumption triggered, rate to what extent you agree that it is true using the following scale:

0. Not at all

1. Somewhat

2. Moderately

3. A Lot

Matthias's rating: 3. A Lot

STEP 5. DISPUTE BY QUESTIONING THE ASSUMPTION IDENTIFIED

Dispute the assumption by questioning its value, logic, fairness, evidence, or accuracy, or all these qualities.

Possible Questions to Ask:

1) What Are The Pluses of Accepting And Those of Rejecting The Assumption?

2) Would I Say it to Someone Else?

3) How Do I Figure?

4) Am I Thinking Rigidly?

5) Am I Labeling?

6) What Are The Exceptions (Search for Exceptions)?

7) Am I Fortune-telling?

8) Am I Catastrophizing?

9) Am I Letting My Feelings Be My Reality?

10) What Would a High-priced Lawyer Say?

Overcoming Disabilities despair

There are various questions that could effectively dispute the helplessness assumption, such as asking about the pluses of accepting or rejecting it and whether you'd say it to someone else (as has been shown with other assumptions), but let's try two new ones and repeat a third just tried in the previous chapter. The three develop their arguments differently: the first by focusing on unfair labeling, the second by looking for needed exceptions, and the third by targeting narrow thinking.

Actual Questions Asked:

Question #5: Am I Labeling?

If you act silly one day at work, do you conclude you're an uncontrollable cutup—a foolish clown? If you forget to put all the ingredients in a recipe you've made seven times before, do you conclude you're a step away from the memory-loss of dementia? If you confuse similar words in a sentence, do you conclude you're muddle-headed? Watch-out for this very human tendency to unfairly label oneself sweepingly after doing something minor, albeit regrettable, once or a few times. It's bullying oneself into despair.

Matthias writes, "I am labeling myself. I'm not helpless because sometimes I ask for help to tie my shoes. Tuesday and Thursday last week I asked for help to do three things. On Monday and Wednesday I didn't ask anyone for help to do anything. I cannot firmly conclude that my actions Tuesday and Thursday mean I'm helpless anymore than my not asking for help Monday and Wednesday definitely mean I'm not helpless. Not asking for help Monday and Wednesday are exceptions to saying I'm helpless (see question #6 below). Some days I need help doing things, other days I don't. I'm no more helpless because of asking for help than stupid because of asking for information."

Question #6: What Are the Exceptions?

Look for instances when assuming your helpless is untrue; they don't fit with the helplessness picture.

Matthias writes "If I'm fatigued, I might need help getting into my scooter, but I still volunteer at the hospital on those days. It may take me a while to prepare dinner, but I do it and do it well. I author stories, am a critical reviewer, can repair almost anything having to do with the telephone, and more. I do lots. I'm far from being helpless."

Question #4: Am I Thinking Rigidly?

Rigid thinking is black and white thinking, all or nothing thinking, success or failure thinking; it overlooks the freeing in-betweens, the shades of gray so necessary to accurate appraisal. Cognitive-behavior therapists observe that categorical thinking (you're good or bad, right or wrong, helpless or helpful) promotes inflexibility and stifles thinking both of which can lead to self-deprecation and despair. Argue against the helplessness assumption by broadening your thinking.

Matthias writes, "Because I need help sometimes, does not mean I need it all times—I'm not helpless. Because I need help with many things does not mean I need it with all things. I might have to call upon the police, the fire department, the paramedics, teachers, even politicians to help me. Needing help and accepting help do not mean helpless."

STEP 6. DISPUTE BY CHALLENGING THE ASSUMPTION IDENTIFIED

Dispute the assumption by challenging behaviorally the part that says, "and there's nothing I can do about it." Make a challenge to that part, refute or cast reasonable doubt on it, by doing something constructive.

Possible Challenges to Make:

1) Challenge by Assertiveness

2) Challenge by Activation

3) Challenge by Problem-solving

4) Challenge by Contracting

5) Challenge by Relaxation

6) Challenge by Exposure

Overcoming Disabilities despair

Actual Challenges Made:

Challenge #3: The Problem-solving Challenge

Problem-solving challenges a misery-making assumption's proclamation that nothing can be done by proving that something can be done. Problem-solving shows what can be done. Matthias's problem is proving he can do something that meaningfully reduces his feelings of vulnerability to assault. Solving this problem will dispute the assumption that disability means helpless, and there's nothing that can be done about it. Here are critical problem-solving steps and how Matthias applies them:

a. State the problem to be solved.

"My problem is I'm easy prey for those who would rob me by breaking into my home; I'm no longer able to fight back effectively."

b. State your goal.

"I want to better protect myself and my family from those who would do us harm."

c. List possible solutions. (Think of as many as you can without worrying whether they are feasible for now — brainstorm)

1) buy a big dog

2) ask Tom Jenkins, my neighbor, to watch my home

3) ask the police to send more patrol cars around my neighborhood

4) become more active in neighborhood watch

5) install an alarm system in my home

d. List probable solutions. (From the list of possible solutions, choose those which are, at this moment, feasible.)

"The three I choose are (1) buy a big dog, (3) more police, (5) alarm system."

e. State probable solution to try first and why.

"I like #5, the alarm system, because it doesn't involve the care and maintenance a dog(#1) would. Also, cops (#3) don't have the personnel to monitor the area as much as I want. So, I like the alarm system best; it's costly though, but I think I can swing it."

f. Name steps required to implement probable solution (i.e., #5).

1. check the phonebook for alarm system companies

2. find out about price and installation

3. ask Tom, Al, and John what alarm systems they like

g. Describe result of trying probable solution (i.e., #5).

"I bought a system. More money than I thought, but I'm happy. Glad a security company monitors it. Also, like fire alarm and panic button features (put one downstairs and one upstairs). More security now, really feel less vulnerable. No need to try any of the other probable solutions I listed."

Sometimes the problem has several parts, each a problem in and of itself. Solve each part to solve the whole. Suppose making dinner is the predicament. Divide the task into its parts: getting recipe, shopping, cooking, and so on, and find a solution for each.

Use problem-solving by itself or combine it with other behavioral challenges like Activation.

STEP 7. REAPPRAISE

Devise a fairer, more helpful way of looking at whatever triggered — incidents, comments, recollections, etc. — the nasty assumption identified. Compare your thinking now with your thinking then. Look at what you said in step three. What would you say now? You may have to think about that for a few days or weeks first.

After Matthias purchased the alarm system, he could write, "Okay, I'm angry at a justice system that pardons those who continue to victimize us. Like anyone else, I too might become a victim, but I can and will take steps to help myself not be. I'm certainly no fighter, so maybe a few more protections is a good idea. Not going to lie down and shiver, going to do something to help myself. I use a cane most of the time and sometimes my hands and knees hurt so bad I don't want to even be touched. Wish they didn't, but sometimes they do. Wish I weren't disabled, but I am. Wish I could do more, but still can do a lot. I'm not helpless.

If I continue assuming RA makes me helpless, and there's nothing I can do about it, I'll stop looking for solutions to the problems I encounter. Better for me to assume that brainstorming makes most problems solvable, and that failing to help myself sometimes does not mean I'll fail to help myself all times...does not mean I'm helpless."

STEP 8. CONSIDER AGAIN THE MISERY-GENERATING ASSUMPTION IDENTIFIED AND RE-RATE HOW MUCH YOU AGREE THAT IT IS TRUE

What do you now say after having questioned and challenged the assumption and reappraised the events triggering it? Apply the scale used in step 4, and compare your responses then with those now. To what extent do you still believe that disability means helpless, and there's nothing you can do about it.

Possible ratings:

0. Not at all

1. Somewhat

2. Moderately

3. A Lot

Matthias's previous rating: #3 A Lot

Matthias's current rating: #0 Not at all

STEP 9. RE-RATE THE STRENGTH OF THE EMOTIONS YOU NAMED PREVIOUSLY

As in step 2, rate from 1 to 100 the degree you feel each emotion. Compare your ratings now with those made before and note the difference, if any.

Matthias's previous ratings: vulnerability (90), fear (70), despair (80), anger (90)

Matthias's current ratings: vulnerability (30), fear (30) despair (10), anger (90)

As Matthias writes, "My feelings of vulnerability, fear, and despair have each lessened dramatically, despair the most. As I continue to show myself I can do things and prove that I'm far from helpless, I hope my feelings of vulnerability and fear will shrink even more. I don't really think that despair will drop further, and I'm not surprised I still feel as angry now as before because I still think the justice system leaves lots to be desired."

Disability does not mean helpless, but before you're convinced, you'll probably have to dispute this assumption several times in several different circumstances. And when you do, perhaps you'll prefer using questions and challenges other than those used here.
Can you be disabled and be strong, independent, self-reliant? Matthias's initial answer to that question, as indicated, would be a resounding no. In time and with practice at disputing disability assumption #4, he should change his mind. My answer to the can you be disabled and strong, etc., question is: absolutely, I know so. I also know that if you believe otherwise, if you believe disability means helpless and you're convinced you're unable to complete tasks that you should be able to complete, or you think you're now a lamb in a world of hungry wolves, or you believe you've become a millstone around the necks of family and friends, you'll be sad, dispirited, and eventually perhaps even clinically depressed.

Matthias is well on the road to liberating himself from assuming disability means helpless. But he still needs to face its frequent companion, namely, disability means hopeless. In next chapter, he does.

CHAPTER 7 Disability assumption #5: Disability Means Hopeless

This chapter continues with Matthias Wilson, showing him applying here what he's previously learned. His goal now is to begin giving up the assumption that disability means hopeless. More questioning tactics are described and what to do when the problem-solving challenge fails is considered.

STEP 1 DESCRIBE WHAT HAPPENED THAT UPSET YOU

Something upset you. Write down what. Possibly nothing specific you can name took place other than just thinking of things — daydreams, recollections, worries about what's to come — and your depressed mood seems to worsen or harden; detail your thoughts

Matthias writes "I'm worried about the tomorrows to come. It helps just to say that. Since the doctor first told me of my sentence, hardly a day goes by that I don't fear the future and feel cheated. Thank God for Elaine and the girls. Otherwise, each time things got worse, it'd be too scary. But after this last little problem my daily down hit a new low and my daily fear a new high. While typing an e-mail to my sister, Marie, my wrist and fingers felt unusually stiff and painful. Used to type 80 words per minute, but lately half that's speedy for me. Now, I'm even less than that. Quit doing the letter. Could have done a little more, just didn't want to."

STEP 2 NAME AND RATE YOUR NEGATIVE FEELINGS

Write down your feelings - name them - and rate how strongly from 1 (hardly at all) to 100 (extremely) you feel them.

After the typing difficulty, Matthias states and rates his feelings as follows: foreboding (70), hopelessness (90), futility (90), despair (80)

STEP 3. IDENTIFY EACH MISERY-GENERATING ASSUMPTION TRIGGERED

Ask yourself why you feel the way you feel. To answer, try to recover the thoughts you had when the situation that upset you happened—replay your inner voice. From those thoughts search for each misery- making assumption triggered. Do each assumption separately.

Matthias's Disabling Thoughts:

Matthias writes, "My first thought was, ' how can this be happening,' which upon reflection led to my next thought, 'I'm soon going to have to give up the typing of those short stories I love to do.' Then I thought, 'guess my window is closing, everything's vanishing. Soon everything will be gone. Nothing will be left. No future. It's only a matter of time, and time isn't on my side.' "

Possible Disability Assumptions:

1) If I'm disabled, my worth is diminished, and there's nothing I can do about it

2) If I'm disabled, I can never be happy again, and there's nothing I can do about it

3) If I'm disabled, I look ugly, and there's nothing I can do about it

4) If I'm disabled, I'm helpless, and there's nothing I can do about it

5) If I'm disabled, I have no hope for the future, and there's nothing I can do about it

Disability Assumption Identified:

Matthias says that the underlying assumption is: "If I have disabling RA, I

have no hope for the future, and there's nothing I can do about it." He continues, "That's not an eye-opener for me; I live with that daily."

Overcoming Disabilities despair

STEP 4. RATE HOW MUCH YOU AGREE THAT THE ASSUMPTION IDENTIFIED IS TRUE

For each assumption triggered, rate to what extent you agree that it is true using the following scale:

0. Not at all

1. Somewhat

2. Moderately

3. A Lot

Matthias's rating is: 3. A Lot *

STEP 5. DISPUTE BY QUESTIONING THE ASSUMPTION IDENTIFIED

Dispute the assumption by questioning its value, logic, fairness, evidence, or accuracy, or all these qualities.

Possible Questions to Ask:

1) What Are The Pluses of Accepting And Those of Rejecting The Assumption?

2) Would I Say it to Someone Else?

3) How Do I Figure?

4) Am I Thinking Rigidly?

5) Am I Labeling?

6) What Are The Exceptions (Search for Exceptions)?

7) Am I Fortune-telling?

8) Am I Catastrophizing?

9) Am I Letting My Feelings Be My Reality?

10) What Would a High-priced Lawyer Say?

Actual Questions Asked:

Question #7. Am I Fortune-telling?

81

After lecturing on a scientific concept, one of my (MDL) professors would always say, "Okay, how do you know?" His goal was challenging students to think critically and not just accept the concept as fact. The same question applies here. "How do you know what's in your future?" You don't. The fortune-telling question is concerned with thinking the worst will happen when in fact something bad may or may not happen.

For this question, Matthias writes, "I think I am fortune-telling, because when I assume hopelessness and bleakness, I'm saying everything in my future looks bad. But RA is, if anything, unpredictable. No one knows for sure when it will do what. Don't know how much joint-function in how many joints I'll lose or how fast I'll lose it. Maybe the medicine, the exercises, my diet, and my attitude will stem the tide appreciably. I don't want to bet the worst will happen; that's betting against myself."

Question #8. Am I Catastrophizing?

Fortune-telling and catastrophizing are cognitive cousins; the fortune-telling forecast of a bleak future becomes the ammunition for catastrophizing. The catastrophizer says that whatever will happen will be so awful that coping with it will be impossible.

Matthias states, "I think I am catastrophizing, because I'm implying that if the worst happens, whatever that will be, I won't be able to handle it. But so far I have been able to handle the pain and stiffness RA causes, so I do deal with things. Sure, there are bad days, but there are good days, too. Guess the really important question is how much disability can I stand. Don't know right now but mustn't forget that my mind (my outlook) and my body are different. There have been many disabled people, some extremely so like the physicist Stephen Hawking and the actor Christopher Reeve, who have kept mind and body separated in order to lead productive and fulfilling lives. There are many others like them living today. I think I can stand much more than I credit myself for. Certainly I don't want to let a sense of hopelessness run my life to ruin."

Question #1. What Are The Pluses Of Accepting and Those of Rejecting The Assumption?

Look closely at the assumption. What does accepting it do for you? What does rejecting it do for you? Do the pluses of rejecting outnumber or outweigh, or both outnumber and outweigh, those of accepting? If the pluses of rejecting are greater, likely they are, you have put into question the assumption's utility for you and by so doing siphoned a bit of its power over you.

Matthias writes, "I really can't see any pluses to accepting the assumption. It depresses me. Pluses of rejecting the assumption are feeling less despair and having a better outlook. I don't know what the future has in store, but I do have a lot going for me now. To feel so depressed all the time, so hopeless and scared all the time, robs me of the mastery, fun, and joy, I can now have. By assuming disability means hopeless, I kind of make it happen. If I believe there's no use, I kind of foreclose on me. I prevent myself from building skills I need to stand-up to this damn disease."

Question # 2. Would I Say it to Someone Else?

What would you tell a friend with RA? Argue against the hopelessness assumption.

Matthias says, "Here's what I would tell another person with RA: give yourself hope, build hope. It's true that you can't do what you used to, but as you age the disease may or may not worsen. If it gets worse, it will be more difficult to do what you can do now. Yet don't forget that many things get harder to do as you get older; able 70-year-olds can't do what they did when 40, but they can do many things. Search for what's manageable that's fulfilling or pleasurable, or ideally that's both fulfilling and pleasurable. Don't hide in a cocoon of fear, worry, sadness, and despair. Don't let the threat of calamity become the calamity."

Question # 9. Am I Letting My Feelings Be My Reality?

It's logical for reality to influence, even define feelings. How you live and what befalls you will greatly affect your emotions. But it's illogical to let feelings define reality—to let how you feel represent what in fact is. Yet that is what numbers of depressed individuals do, a misery-making style of thinking that, as said, many cognitive behavior therapists call emotional reasoning.

Matthias writes, "When I let how I feel (hopeless), tell me things are hopeless, I'm saying how I feel is how things are. But how I feel is not necessarily the true picture of reality. If I feel dumb for making a mistake, am I really dumb, dumb to all who know me? Feeling a sense of hopelessness doesn't mean things actually are hopeless in every way, every day forever. It's important I separate feelings from facts and not foreclose on myself with feelings that stop me from coping."

STEP 6 DISPUTE BY CHALLENGING THE ASSUMPTION IDENTIFIED

Dispute the assumption by challenging behaviorally the part that says, "and there's nothing I can do about it." Make a challenge to that part, refute or cast reasonable doubt on it, by doing something constructive.

Possible Challenges to Make:

1) Challenge by Assertiveness

2) Challenge by Activation

3) Challenge by Problem-solving

4) Challenge by Contracting

5) Challenge by Relaxation

6) Challenge by Exposure

Actual Challenges Made:

Challenge #3. The Problem-solving Challenge

As a challenge to a misery-generating assumption's proclamation that nothing can be done, problem-solving shows what can be done. By proving that you can cope with new difficulties, problem-solving, as used here, casts doubt on the idea that you won't be able to deal with the future; in so doing, problem-solving drains some of the fear from the nagging question: "What will I do if...?" Problem-solving steps and Matthias's comments follow:

a. State the problem to be solved.

"What would I do if I could no longer type? How would I write the stories I love to create?"

b. State your goal.

"To be able to finish the stories I want to finish."

c. List possible solutions. (Think of as many as you can without worrying whether they are feasible.)

1) dictate stories to a typist

2) dictate stories onto a tape and have a secretary transcribe them

3) use speech recognition software with my computer to minimize keystroking

d. List probable solutions. (From the list of possible solutions, choose those which are, at this moment, feasible.)

2. taping dictation and having it transcribed

3. speech recognition software

e. State probable solution to try first and why.

"Number 2. I like the dictation idea and having someone else transcribe the tape. It's simple and still gives me control over what I want to say. I can change the tape as much as I want before having it typed."

f. Name steps required to implement #2:

1) Borrow a dictating machine and tape from Pat, who I know still uses one at his work.

2) Practice. See if I can dictate a story, one from something I've typed and another from just sitting and thinking about what I want to say.

3) Hire a typist from the community newspaper who will work cheaply.

g. Describe result of trying probable solution (i.e., #2).

"Things didn't go as I'd hoped. The dictating went okay, but it's is impossible to revise right away when you can't see what you've said right away.

The typist was inexpensive, but long projects would get pricey. Also, I wasn't all that happy with her accuracy and with having a stranger in my home. This could be a solution, but there are better ones for me, so I'll try another."

h. Probable solution to try second. Number 3.

"I'd like to try the speech recognition software idea. Eliminates need for typist. Gives me more independence. But biggest plus, if it works, is immediately seeing what I've done and being able to revise on the spot. Mark swears by it—uses it a lot and loves it. Comparatively cheap, and if it happens that I can no longer type, it's a viable alternative."

I. Steps required to implement #3:

4) talk to Mark about what he has, and what I require, computer memory, etc.

5) phone the stores, get prices

6) select, purchase, and have delivered

7) learn & practice the technology now

j. Result of trying #3.

"Bingo! Did all the steps. System works really well. Practice will make it even better. Slowly, I'm becoming less dependent on the keyboard and the mouse—love to kill that creature. Don't need the software for everything now, hope I never will need it for everything, but nice to know it's there and that I can use it effectively, actually like it. Intend to use it right away for some things. This exercise helps prove to me in a very real way that I can handle problems RA brings. Need not feel so scared and hopeless about the future."

STEP 7. REAPPRAISE

Devise a fairer, more helpful way of looking at whatever triggered— incidents, comments, recollections, etc.—the nasty assumption identified. Compare your thinking now with your thinking then. Look at what you said in step three. What would you say now? You may have to think about that for a few days or weeks first.

After a few days of thinking things over, Matthias said, "It's like there's two of us in one body. There's the me who experiences every change, and there's the me, the doomsayer-judge, who watches, watches, and watches. And waits for the worst. I experienced lots of pain in my fingers and wrist so I couldn't type easily, and the doomsayer-judge said, 'See I was waiting for something like that. It's over. You're through. Give it up.' And so I did, then.

My typing took a downturn. Maybe it's permanent, maybe it's not, probably it's not. If it is permanent, however, I'll find another way to do the writing that sharpens, motivates, and energizes me. Whatever happens, I can't let the doomsayer run me, ruin me. He drains me, stopping me from even wanting to try to cope. Can't quit. Won't quit. Quitting finishes you."

STEP 8. CONSIDER AGAIN THE MISERY-GENERATING ASSUMPTION IDENTIFIED AND RE-RATE HOW MUCH YOU AGREE THAT IT IS TRUE

What do you now say after having questioned and challenged the assumption and reappraised the events triggering it? Apply the scale used in step 4, and compare your responses then with those now. To what extent do you still believe that disability means hopeless, and there's nothing you can do about it.

Possible ratings:

0. Not at all

1. Somewhat

2. Moderately

3. A Lot

Matthias's previous rating: #3 A Lot

Matthias's current rating: #2 Moderately

STEP 9. RE-RATE THE STRENGTH OF THE EMOTIONS YOU NAMED PREVIOUSLY

As in step 2, rate from 1 to 100 the degree you feel each emotion. Compare your ratings now with those made before and note the difference, if any.

Matthias's previous ratings: foreboding (70), hopelessness (90), futility (90), despair (80) Matthias's current ratings: foreboding (50), hopelessness (30), futility (30), despair (20)

Matthias writes, "My negative feelings of foreboding dropped by 20 and hopelessness, futility, and despair by 60 each. But I know I need more than just finding a different way to type my stories to rid myself of these destructive feelings. Some amount of fear about the future is with me every day. I accept that. It's reasonable. How could anyone with a chronic degenerative disease like RA not worry about the future? But what the exercises on helplessness and hopelessness did and repeating them when needed will continue to do is help me better control the destructive feelings these helpless and hopeless disability assumptions generate, feelings crippling my motivation to cope with RA."

As the previous five chapters show, the algorithm is applicable to an array of disabling conditions resulting in disabilities despair. When applying the algorithm to a specific incident, event, or situation be mindful that days or weeks may elapse before the algorithm begins to have its intended effects; in particular, it may take a while before the arguments you advance when questioning an assumption begin to resonate with you and the challenges you devise to disprove it begin to bear fruit. Disabilities despair can be stubborn.

So, be patient and be perseverant. Talk away what's getting you down each time something happens to get you down. Identify the misery-making assumptions behind the despair and dispute them with personally meaningful questions, arguments, and challenges.

Overcoming Disabilities despair

Repeat this process until you free yourself from the crushing grip of assuming the worst.

The questions and challenges—the CBT tools— for disputing assumptions are flexible. Chapter 9 summarizes the tools that have been exemplified and introduces two new challenges, mentioned but not as yet discussed. Next, however, we'll look at three side-effects of disability commonly experienced by many of the disabled.

Overcoming Disabilities despair

CHAPTER 8 Disability Fallout

Comparing before you were disabled to now, answer these questions about three often reported disability side effects:

Have you much less energy, that is, fatigue more easily now?

Is it harder to get a good night's sleep now?

Are your relationships with loved ones strained or more strained now?

If you answered yes to any of these questions, this chapter is for you. It offers tips to help you manage fatigue, improve sleep, and get along better with those you love.

Fatigue:

Energy is the blood of life, so no wonder feeling tired and sapped within a few hours after arising is so depressing. Such excessive and unexplainable fatigue is common among many of the disabled and can be serious enough to prevent some from continuing to work; disability fatigue, for want of a better name for this energy vacuum, is one of the most frequent complaints of those with multiple sclerosis. It truly is, I can attest, awful. Whereas normal fatigue follows arduous or extended activity, disability fatigue occurs anytime and everywhere. It allows for little reprieve. According to the Multiple Sclerosis Council of America, such fatigue depletes you so much that you'll feel you haven't the physical or mental strength to do even basic tasks. It's still a mystery why some disabled have it worse than others do or, most important, how to get rid of it, but we can suggest these ways to lessen disability fatigue:

1. Activate, Don't Over-activate

Exercise prudently. Avoid killer aerobics in favor of mild to moderate aerobics; do this less strenuous kind 3 to 5 times a week for about 30 minutes each time. Alternatively or additionally if able, do regular calisthenics and lift lightweights; both will help you stay fit and forestall the muscle weakness that contributes to fatigue. But know your limits. Tailor what and how much you do to fit your needs and capabilities.

Strive to become a wiser steward of your energy. Occupational therapists can help you do that by teaching you ENERGY EFFECTIVENESS. Practising it will allow you to work and play smarter to save energy.

2. Nap

When I was a youngster, my surgeon-grandfather taught me the wonders of napping. Arising daily at 6:00 a.m. for hospital-rounds and surgery, he would return home about noon for one of my grandmother's elaborate full-course lunches—fancy dinners to anyone else—after which he'd head for his study and easy-chair to enjoy a brief snooze. Anyone foolish enough to disturb him would soon regret doing so; napping he absolutely had to do for his own health and that of his patients.

Twenty minutes sufficed for him; ten minutes usually is all I need. After two hours in front of a classroom of 100 college undergraduates, a 10-20 minute shutdown revitalizes me for the rest of the day. An indulgence, no. An essential, yes.

3. Stay Cool

Heat and humidity, yuck! Indeed, as little as a half a degree jump in temperature will make some MS sufferers feel weaker. If heat fatigues you, whatever your disability, try cooler drinks---iced tea rather than hot tea, iced coffee rather than hot coffee---and take cooler showers.

Likewise, avoid long periods in hot humid rooms. Either don't go there or, as the student in the following example did for me because I had to be there, cool the room down. One June day, I was scheduled to supervise the therapy-work of a young woman in a our clinical psychology program. Although the day was pleasant, the room was not; it was stifling. As soon as I push-rolled into it to watch videotapes and discuss cases, I knew I had to get out; the temperature must have been 85 degrees in there. I told the student I couldn't last. So, to cool the room, she proposed running a fan she would borrow from our upstairs clinic. Skeptical, I nonetheless thanked her and agreed to her plan. Five minutes later, she plugged in the fan and 20 minutes after that I felt 200% better. I now own a fan like it and, even in my air-conditioned home, use it to cool my office still more on particularly humid days.

4. Relax

Stress aggravates disability in many ways one of which is by interfering with sleep, a disruption exacerbating fatigue. Relaxation will be discussed in the next chapter.

5. Consider "Anti-fatigue" Medicines

Talk to your doctor. Two main drugs for chronic disability fatigue, often taken by those with multiple sclerosis, are, Amantadine and Pemoline. Amantadine significantly helps about 20% to 40% of the mildly to moderately disabled, but researchers don't know how it works. Pemoline, a central nervous system stimulant, is sometimes effective for those unresponsive to Amantadine. Others to try if these fail you include Modafinil (Alertec), which counters the sleep attacks of narcolepsy, and Ritalin, which stimulates the central nervous system; Ritalin is often prescribed for hyperactivity and attention deficit disorder.

Alas, there as yet is no "silver bullet" for eliminating disability fatigue for all the disabled, but new drugs are on the horizon.

6. Sleep Well

Easier said than done. The next section of this chapter discusses sleep, so I won't say more here.

Which fatigue management strategies are best for you, no one but you can say. Find out. Experiment. Your goal is not to eliminate disability fatigue, unlikely anyway, but to control it better. While trying to do that, be optimistic and keep informed. And be cautious—more out there will disappoint than delight.

Sleep and Sleep Troubles

"Just forgive him. Ray was under lots of pressure. He made a mistake. No reason to kick him out, I implored, but they disagreed."

And like a kid denied a toy, Bruce Perry felt like crying.

"I didn't get my way, a 50-year-old baby, I guess. Tears welled-up inside me, but thank heavens my eyes stayed dry."

All this happened to instructor Bruce Perry at a departmental meeting about Raymond, a student he liked, but actually not all that much. What upset Bruce was being overruled.

"Had to leave the room before my emotional dam burst," he said.

Bruce's back had been keeping him up nightly for hours, nights on end. His uncustomary fragility at the meeting was likely due to his prolonged sleep deprivation.

You sleep, even if only briefly and fitfully; endless nights without would be deadly. Normal sleep, according to the fourth edition of the Diagnostics and Statistics Manual of the American Psychiatric Association (DSM 4), proceeds through five distinct stages: rapid eye movement (REM), which is the stage where dreams occur, and four non-REM stages.

REM accounts for 20 to 25 percent of total sleep time and happens cyclically throughout the night about once every 80 to 100 minutes.

Stage 1, falling from wakefulness to sleep, lasts approximately 5% of the total sleep time.

Stage 2 lasts around 50 percent.

Stages 3 and 4 (deep sleep) comprise from 10 to 20 percent.

All this happens nightly—if everything goes as it should. But too often not everything does go as it should, which is why few of us beyond our teen years can boast never having had a sleepless night.

So, what ruins sleep for so many? Lots can. Stress, worry, pain, even mild discomfort are a few of the intruders that can keep you up. As well, crossing time zones and working night-shifts can zombify your body and petrify your mind. Changing time zones rapidly, which causes jet lag, and working nights/sleeping days (night shifts) confuse the circadian rhythm—the inborn biological rhythm making you want to sleep when it's dark and awaken when it's light. The over-the-counter drug melatonin may help mitigate circadian problems. (The brain naturally produces melatonin during the dark hours, stopping production when it gets light.)

Another sleep-wrecker for many, a decidedly upsetting one, is obstructive sleep apnea--- episodes of no breathing. It's a common breathing-related sleep disorder that arises when, during sleep, the normal constriction of the upper airway muscles becomes excessive. Too much constriction causes the apnea. The unlucky person with obstructive sleep apnea, usually a middle-aged overweight male, may be unaware he has it. But his bed partner will be painfully aware, kept awake by the man's loud snoring and ominous---though thankfully brief---periods of no breathing followed by jolting snores when breathing resumes. Special doctor-prescribed breathing devices worn during sleep can help alleviate the problem.

TROUBLESHOOTING THE SLEEP TROUBLES

If you think your sleeping problems are breathing related, ask your doctor for a referral to a sleep specialist. The doctor may first, however, suggest sleeping pills, perhaps benzodiazepines, to give you more immediate relief from sleeplessness. But be careful when taking them: if used continually, you'll likely become dependent on them. Then, after stopping, there's a good chance the insomnia will return with even worse symptoms. So what can one do to help oneself sleep better? There are 11 things. Most of them are based on a seemingly commonsensical psychological principle called stimulus control.

Several years ago, two days before the final exam in my class on abnormal psychology, a student with bloodshot eyes, mussed hair, and sweaty brow knocked loudly on my office door and pleaded:

"I want to go to Psych. grad school. Please know I can do better than what I'm getting in your class."

"What's the problem?" I wanted to help.

"I can't seem to study well this term. I just moved into the University Dorm. I always fall asleep whenever I study there."

He sounded desperate. "How do you study?," I asked.

"Three days before each of your tests, I try to cram six hours straight, a night. I study after dinner. The library on campus is a zoo in the evening, so I stay in my dorm room. My roomy's quiet, but the dorm's noisy."

"How is it that you fall asleep? Do you fall asleep at your desk?"

"I guess the material bores me." I took no offense. "I don't like my desk; the chair's too hard; I study in bed. Why can't I study better?"

I knew why, though I didn't say right away. His problem was bad stimulus control. He did his studying after dinner in bed, probably tired, and just before the test which forced him to tackle too much in too little time. He needed to stop cramming and instead spread his studying over more days; he needed to study before he filled his stomach and became sleepy; he needed to study where he didn't customarily nod off. He needed to rearrange his world so that the right conditions for the behavior he wanted to occur did occur. In short, he needed better stimulus control, as regards studying.

Maybe you need better stimulus control, as regards sleeping. If so, follow this straightforward sleep-better advice of sleep experts like Drs. Richard Bootzin, Robert Leahy, Stephen Holland, and S. Scholcket:

1. Go to bed only when sleepy.

2. Get up at night if not sleepy.

If you can't fall asleep for what seems to be about 15 to 20 minutes, get up and go to another room. Come back to the bedroom only when sleepy. You may have to repeat this several times a night for a while.

3. Get up in the morning at about the same time, seven days a week.

Set the alarm and obey it no matter how lousy your night's sleep. Eventually an effective pattern will emerge.

4. Keep the bed pure.

Don't use the bed for anything but sleeping—no reading, no eating, no TV, no worrying; write down the worries and question them when out of the bedroom. Make the bed the place to sleep, and that's all it's for. Okay, concur the experts, there's one exception, and that's sex.

Overcoming Disabilities despair

5. Limit caffeine.

Numbers of us punctuate our lives with coffee, tea, or caffeinated-cola. Having too many of these and other similar stimulants will exact an unwelcome nightly price, as my friend and colleague found out.

"I haven't had a good night sleep in five years," he said. "I'm up four times a night and have a hell of the time falling back asleep. I'd give anything to change that. I'm a zombie the next day."

I asked whether he brought home his worries, and he said no. So we explored his habits and found that each evening he downed two cups of Cappuccino.

"Cut out the nighttime exotic coffee," I advised.

He protested, "But I need that."

I guess he had shallow limits to how much he'd sacrifice. However, that soon changed. After a few more sleep-disturbed nights, he stopped the nightly caffeine-fix and slept well.

6. Build a good sleep environment.

Your room should be reasonably quiet and the temperature and mattress comfortable.

7. Limit booze.

Make sure there are at least four hours between your last shot and when your head hits the pillow. True, a little bit of alcohol may cause drowsiness, but it may also disrupt REM sleep---dream time---which could exacerbate your feelings of fatigue the next day.

8. Relax before going to bed.

If tension keeps you up, perhaps you bring the stress of your job into your bedroom, relaxation, which will be described in the next chapter, may help you sleep.

9. No napping

Napping fights fatigue, as noted, so let's amend no napping to no over 30 minutes late afternoon or evening napping.

10. Don't exercise strenuously during the two hours before bed.

11. Don't retire thirsty or hungry.

But, to minimize urinary urgencies, I advise not to load up on liquids.

Sleep better, feel better.

Relating

My center is the relationship I have with my wife, which over the years has weathered philosophical, financial, and career challenges. Now it struggles with my unstoppable MS. If your relationship with spouse or partner is hurting, listen closely to how you talk to one another. Distrust, animosity, rejection, misunderstanding, and defensiveness all thrive in the soil of destructive communication.

TALKING TURN-OFFS

In Leader Effectiveness Training, Dr. Thomas Gordon identifies these ways we pollute the communication soil:

- Blaming. "It's your fault for not...."

- Interrogating. "Tell me again step-by-step how you could let that happen."

- Shaming, name-calling, and ridiculing. "Did you see the look on their faces when you said that to Marty? Really, you sure were a jerk tonight."

- Ordering and commanding. "Don't ever let that happen again."

- Preaching. "We all have our jobs. It's yours to.... That's just how it is."

- Interpreting. "You did that because you have an...."

- Threatening. "If you don't... there'll be hell to pay."

- Lecturing. "Listen carefully. I'll explain each step precisely. First...."

- Minimizing---my addition to the list. "You think you're tired and achy. You don't know what tired and achy really is. Let me tell you about the fatigue I suffer."

The turn-offs hammer partners and either intentionally or unintentionally demean, deny, and detract. They're sometimes delivered aggressively or condescendingly or indignantly or moralistically, but they're always delivered insensitively. None builds trust, shows caring, or strengthens bonds. Turn off the turn-offs.

TALKING TURN-ONS

Help your partner feel accepted and safe, so he or she will open up to you. Cultivate the communication soil. Here are a few ways to enrich it:

Speak with "I's"

If you want Joanna to know your viewpoint and not get defensive if it questions hers, reveal it with "I" statements.

"Joanna, I feel hurt when I'm left out of your plans."

The alternative is to you her.

"Joanna, you're rude to leave me out of your plans."

"I" statements further communication. "You" ones stop it, especially when they accuse, blame, or shame; really upsetting ones will likely make your partner defensive or want to retaliate. It's impossible to never say "you", but rather than saying what's wrong with your partner, use "I" to explain how you feel and how you see things. That helps promote good deep talking.

Show You Value Your Partner: Listen and Tune in

Priceless in revealing your listening and want to understand are:

- Rephrasing what your partner says by repeating back the phrases you hear

- Inquiring when you don't understand

- Keeping eye contact to demonstrate that you are paying attention

- Validating your partner by saying you agree with what's been said, when you honestly do agree

Overcoming Disabilities despair

Conversations die when the listener responds with irrelevant questions, nonsensical comments, or disinterest.

For instance, your partner, tears in her eyes, tells you how difficult her day has been, and you say:

"Did you see how bright the sun was this afternoon?"

Likewise, conversations die when the listener interprets and blames:

"Well, Mark, you clearly have made a mistake."

And they have short lives when the listener preaches and lectures:

"If you want to avoid problems like that in the future, do this one simple thing: find out ahead of time what all the criteria are."

Conversely, talks enliven when the listener shows understanding, interest, and attention:

"Sarah, correct me if I'm wrong, but I think you're saying that it hurts when someone like Mary criticizes your work and, if I have it right, that you see advantages to changing positions."

Show You Value Your Partner: Encourage Talking

Says marriage therapist Laurie Cope Grand, in *The Marriage & Family Presentation Guide*, open-ended questions promote talking.

Your partner, Linda, tells you of overhearing her co-worker, Robert , criticizing her financial report, which took her hours to complete the evening before. If you ask her, "How do you feel about what Robert said?", your open-ended question encourages her to continue sharing. It does not request a yes or no response; it asks her to reflect on her emotions — the heart of her message.

An open-ended question that's a talk-initiator might be:

"How was your day?"

So also might be:

"What do you think about continuing to work there? "

More focused, but still a talk--stimulator is the request for details:

"Linda, tell me what are the advantages in your mind for keeping that job?"

Show You Value Your Partner: Listen Empathically & Solve Problems Together

Create a warm safe environment where you and your partner build bridges not fences. That's an environment of understanding, sincerity, genuineness, and mutual regard. It's an environment where both of you listen empathically to each other, trying to understand how the other feels and sees things.

It's also an environment where you seek solutions together, even to small problems; many times it's the small ones that irreparably damage the relationship. Here are two versions of Paul and Amy trying to solve a small problem. After Paul, diagnosed with a severe case of untreated Lyme's disease several years ago and now reliant upon a cane, and Amy speak, I'll say what each has done.

Accusatory, Destructive Version:

Paul says, "Amy, do you realize we're out of vitamins again? Why didn't you pick them up when you went shopping? Tell me why?" (Interrogating, attempting to shame)

Amy says, "You didn't tell me they were gone. I'm not psychic. I had to buy lots of stuff, and vitamins just weren't on my mind." (Blaming, defending).

Paul says, "But it's up to you to buy them. Think about how important it is for me to get proper nutrition. You know what the doctor said." (Blaming, preaching, lecturing, attempting to shame)

Amy says, "Get off my back, Paul. Can't you realize how tired work makes me. If you want them so bad, get off the couch and get them yourself. Maybe that should be your job. I do most of the shopping. Correction, I do all the shopping." (Ordering, ridiculing, threatening, shaming)

Paul says, "You're being mean, Amy. You know it's hard for me to get around. Going to the store would sap all my energy. You really don't know what tired is. If you did, you wouldn't say such dumb things. I do lots of stuff for you that uses up lots of my energy. Is that what you want?" (Name-calling, shaming, preaching, minimizing)

Amy says, "There you go again. Making me a villain. Can't you think of anything else to call me? For somebody who's supposed to be smart, you sure have a small vocabulary. I think you want me to be the villain because it makes you feel good. I don't get you vitamins, so I don't care about you." (Name-calling, interpreting, ridiculing)

Understanding, Constructive Version:

Paul says, Amy, it seems like we're out of vitamins. I know you just went shopping. I'm sorry, I should've looked before you left, but I guess I got preoccupied. (Uses "I" statements to accept responsibility for the problem, validates her efforts)

Amy says, "I didn't see they were gone either. I know you need them honey, but I'm really beat right now, all that shopping you know, so can it wait for a bit?" (Shares responsibility, demonstrates concern and interest in his welfare and recognizes his needs, uses "I" statements to describe her feelings)

Paul says, "I'd be tired too if I did all that. What do you think about my calling the pharmacy to have the pills delivered? I don't think it'll cost much, and it'll certainly save going back." (Again validates her efforts and feelings, demonstrates he's concerned and interested, suggests a solution and inquires about it)

Amy says, Great. (Validates his efforts to find a solution)

Version 2 beats version 1 — clearly. No animosity, no name-calling, no fences between them. Amy and Paul join together to solve a problem in a way that, instead of loosening the relationship, tightens it.

Speak well and listen well. Practice the turn-ons, avoid the turn-offs. To strengthen the relationship-bonds, be genuine, sincere, honest, loving, and respecting, and communicate care and concern. Strive to create a climate of acceptance, understanding, openness, and trust so that communication flourishes. That is not easy. But it can be done.

Whatever the disability fallout is for you, by all means seek total solutions to it, but be willing to settle for partial improvements.

CHAPTER 9 A Closer Look Inside Your CBT Toolbox

Most cognitive behavior therapy (CBT) tools in our program of laying waste to destructive disability assumptions are questions and challenges aimed at helping you feel better. Question each assumption's illogic, unfairness, or inadequacy. Challenge each assumption's anti-coping pronouncement. The questions and challenges offer perspective, clarity, and hope.

Questions

Overcoming Disabilities Despair includes 10 questions to help you dispute the disability assumptions. If others or specific modifications of the 10 resonate more with you, use them. Below are summaries of the 10 applied in previous chapters and where in the book you'll find them. When you employ them, devise your own scripts — written arguments. Your arguments are the ones most likely to strike a chord within you, make the most sense to you, and be the ones most likely to work.

1. What Are the Pluses of Accepting and Those of Rejecting the Assumption?

Look closely at the assumption. What does accepting it do for you? What does rejecting it do for you? Do the pluses of rejecting outnumber or outweigh, or both outnumber and outweigh, those of accepting? If they do, likely they do, you have questioned the assumption's utility for you and by so doing siphoned a bit of its power over your feelings and actions. (Examples in chapters 3, 4, 7.)

2. Would You Say it to Someone Else?

Harder on yourself than on others? If you are, ask why the double standard, one for you and one for the rest of us, and the unfairness of what you're doing cries out. (Examples in chapters 3, 4, 5.)

3. How Do You Figure?

Is what you're telling yourself logical? Are you really unworthy if somebody ignores you? Ask yourself (a) if the evidence for what you're telling yourself is solid and (b) if what you're telling yourself is logical. (Example in chapter 3.)

4. Am I Thinking Rigidly?

Good or bad. Ugly or beautiful. Terrible or wonderful. Black or white. All or none. Where are the in-betweens, the gradations, the shades of gray so necessary for clarity, accuracy, breadth? Thinking in either/or categories is thinking rigidly, narrowly, brittlely, and doing so promotes inflexibility, stifles thought, and highlights despair. Find out if you do this. (Example in chapter 6.)

5. Am I Labeling?

Now and forever helpless, if you ask for help with something? Now and forever stupid, if you ask for information? Question how often you label yourself with an all-encompassing, never-ending, no-give nasty. Watch-out for the tendency to unfairly label yourself sweepingly after doing something minor, albeit regrettable. (Example in chapter 6)

6. What Are the Exceptions?

You say you are helpless, useless, whatever, but are you always so? Are you never helpful or useful? To add some healthy, reasonable, liberating doubt to the assumptions depressing you, find the exceptions to them in your life. (Example in chapters 6.)

7. Am I Fortune-telling ?

Predicting a bleak future? Understandably, those saddled with a progressively disabling chronic condition envision the worst. But, as we know, the course of disabling disease is often variable and unpredictable. So, forecasting the ghastliest of outcomes is uncalled for. It's also self-fulfilling if it depresses and drains away your motivation to even try to cope. (Example in chapter 7.)

8. Am I Catastrophizing?

Fortune-telling and catastrophizing are cognitive cousins; the forecast of a bleak future becomes the ammunition for catastrophizing. The catastrophizer says that whatever will happen will be so awful that coping with it will be impossible. (Example in chapter 7.)

9. Am I Letting My Feelings Be My Reality?

Are you saying that because you feel a certain way---helpless or hopeless—you actually are that way? If you do, you are defining reality in terms of feelings. It's logical for reality to influence, even define feelings because what happens to you will greatly affect your emotions. But it's illogical to let feelings define reality—to let how you feel represent what in fact is. Yet that is what numbers of depressed individuals do, a misery-generating style of thinking that many cognitive behavior therapists call emotional reasoning. (Examples in chapters 5, 7.)

10. What Would A High-priced Lawyer Say?

Sometimes it is difficult to argue on your own behalf against a misery-generating assumption because it strikes an especially hard to dispute chord within you. Before giving up, try stepping outside yourself to gain perspective. Imagine you are a lawyer in a courtroom. Cross-examine the believer of the assumption(yourself) about what it proclaims as truth. The lawyer's goal is to inject reasonable doubt into the assumption's proclamations. What does the assumption say? What does it imply? (Example in chapter 4.)

Challenges

Challenges aim to contradict the crippling "there's nothing I can do about it" part of disability assumptions, showing instead that there are things you can do. Four challenges of the six challenges have been exemplified; the two remaining are described here. As with the questioning tools, however, other challenges are certainly possible.

1. Assertiveness

Neither passive nor aggressive, assertive means standing-up for your rights without trampling those of others. Say "I feel" not "you make me feel." "I" statements describe and explain, whereas "you make me" statements accuse. Deliver assertive messages calmly, confidently, respectfully. We have used the assertive challenge to contradict assumption no. 1, disability diminishes worth, but surely it has a wider range. Assertiveness, however, is not the medicine for bettering every human interaction; indeed sometimes the assertive way is the wrong way — don't try it with a raging or abusive person. Be assertive with reasonable people to help them understand your feelings, hear your issues, and respect your position. (Example in chapter 3.)

2. Activation

Do more, feel better. Boost your pleasure or sense of accomplishment, or both, by increasing your activity life. Make certain that the activities chosen are not just boredom-killers, for ultimately these lower mood. The activation challenge works best when plans are detailed and recorded. First, for about a week, take a baseline on how active you are, rating how pleasurable each activity was and how much mastery you felt from doing it. Then, using the same rating system, activate: plan more activity. In doing so, focus your attention on lifters — activities giving you a sense of mastery or pleasure or both. Finally, as soon as convenient after completing a planned activity, record doing it and its actual yield in pleasure and mastery. Proceed slowly but do more and more while keeping mindful of both any roadblocks interfering with your activation goals and ways to remove these obstacles. (Example in chapter 4.)

3. Problem-solving

Like activation, problem-solving gets you going and is a way of coping; the two challenges can work nicely in combination. Problem-solving has several steps:

a. State the problem to be solved.

b. State your goal.

c. List possible solutions. (Think of as many as you can without worrying whether they are feasible, for now — brainstorm)

d. List probable solutions. (From the list of possible solutions, choose those which are, at this moment, feasible.)

e. State probable solution to try first and why.

f. Name steps required to implement probable solution

g. Describe result of trying probable solution

Solve the problem all at once or break it down into its parts, solving each in turn. We have used problem-solving to challenge the assumptions of helplessness and hopelessness, but certainly there are other places for it, too. (Examples in chapter 6,7.)

4. Contracting

Contracting is a system for giving and taking away positives (rewards) for keeping and breaking promises. It's an excellent way to keep motivation high and make a self-improvement program work. As stated in chapter 5, the contract is best when written. It articulates the promises to be kept, the rewards for keeping them, and the consequences for failing to do so. One great strength of the contract is that everything in it is completely spelled out—nothing is vague. A contract can help you activate, be assertive, lose weight, and much much more. It can help you be the best that you can be intellectually, socially, and physically, and in so doing dispute the negativity in a disability assumption.(Example in chapter 5.)

The contract's fuel is the reward, the positive, it uses. For contracts to work well, rewards should be strong and applied contingently and consistently. Rewards are strong when they are things that you desire like clothes, computer equipment, etc. Applying rewards contingently and consistently means living up to each occurrence of the explicit relationship created between the changes desired and the consequences promised. Ally in chapter 5 said that if she didn't snack on candy kisses during the day and evening she would get 1 point towards the purchase of new clothes. Ally clearly stated what gets what and consistently rewarded herself as soon as possible after having lived up to her promise. The points were interim rewards backed up by the true rewards, namely clothes, that they were eventually exchanged for.

Contracts generally work better when the rewards fueling them are not just opportunities to do something desirable that would ordinarily be available were it not for the contract. So, for example, don't back up your earned points only with opportunities to watch certain programs on television that before the contract you would regularly watch or with opportunities to go to plays, concerts, movies, etc., if these are events you previously would go to but are now depriving yourself of for the sake of the contract. Some favorite activities can be set aside as rewards, just don't make all the rewards these kinds of positives.

Giving yourself positives for improving yourself is no more a bribe than is paying a painter for painting your house or receiving a salary for working a week. As Webster defines it, bribery is inducing someone to behave dishonestly or wrongly, is perverting judgment, is corrupting conduct. That's certainly not what you're doing when rewarding yourself to improve yourself.

The two remaining challenges, neither as yet exemplified in the book, are relaxation and exposure. Each can be used alone or combined with one or more of the other challenges. Relaxation is particularly useful for reducing the worry and stress disability assumptions can generate and exposure is particularly useful in modifying fears.

5. Relaxation

Worrying about what the future will bring can cause stress which aggravates multiple sclerosis, rheumatoid arthritis, spinal cord injuries, and similar disabling conditions. Worrying can be mitigated and managed using relaxation.

To experience the sensation of relaxation says Dr. Edmund Jacobson in his classic *Progressive Relaxation*, people must learn the skills of tensing and releasing tension in their muscles. Elaborate and time-consuming, Jacobson's method is nonetheless well worth mastering; variants of it abound in books and tapes.

In *Treatment Plans and Interventions for Depression and Anxiety Disorders*, Drs. Leahy and Holland describe the following three simpler ways to relax, each based on special ways to breathe:

(a) Breathing rhythmically for several minutes. Mouth closed, breathe-in through the nose while counting to six or somewhat less if you prefer. Then, counting the same way, exhale through the nose.

(b) Breath-holding. Again, breathe-in through the nose. This time, however, hold your breath to a three-count. Then, exhale through the mouth.

(c) Breath-counting. This is a form of meditation. Sit comfortably, advise Leahy and Holland, and focus on the floor a "yard or two in front of you." As you breathe through the nose, silently count exhalations from 1 to 10 for up to 15 minutes; 1 to 2 minutes often suffices.

No matter which relaxation exercise you choose, make sure you breathe with your diaphragm when you try it. Diaphragm breathing, the diaphragm is just below the lungs, is breathing as if asleep: breathe-in and the stomach fills with air; breathe-out the stomach flattens. Master the skill of breathing with your diaphragm before attempting any of the three relaxation methods.

6. Exposure

At the age of seven, if given a choice, I'd (MDL) sooner have chewed a worm than pet a dog. No, my appetites weren't strange; I just feared everything canine. My parents once invited a friend to dinner who brought a dog no bigger than a minute. At the sight of it, I hid in the nearest closet — much to my parents chagrin, I'm sure. Don't know why such four-legged creatures affected me so; possibly a dog scared me when I was little, but that's just a guess.

As to why the fear left me, however, I am more certain. When I was 10 years old, my family moved next door to a family that kept large dogs, and for a time my nightmare became my reality. If possible, I'd walk a block out of my way just to avoid seeing their fenced-in beasts. One day, however, the owner invited me to pet his friendliest dog. Without hesitation, I declined. He persisted, and pointing to the black Lab said, "Just hold my hand and let him smell you through the fence." Again, I declined. But he insisted. His persistence tempered with kindness and a promise not to let the dog out emboldened me; so, butterflies wildly flapping in my stomach, I gave it a try. Success. I felt brave, truly wonderful, and bragged to my parents who praised me copiously. The next day I did it again and soon could venture inside the yard to pet the dog. What an achievement. I still don't like unfamiliar dogs, but my urge to run from every pooch that crosses my path no longer rules.

Small, safe, manageable doses of exposure to my fear helped rid me of my fear because it forced me to stop avoiding dogs. Avoidance feeds fear. Exposure starves it, until it's weak or dead. Use exposure to overcome debilitating fears and expected embarrassments. Here's what to do:

(A) Identify The Fear

Maybe for you, fear is looking helpless, different, or feeble. You believe that's what would happen if you were to be seen in a wheelchair, especially at the local mall. The thought doesn't send shivers down your spine but does create enough discomfort to seriously curtail your choices when attempting activation; you tell yourself a walker is bad, but a wheelchair crosses the line. So, to your detriment, you avoid the potential mastery and pleasure experiences of clothes-shopping at the mall because the energy they'd require would force you to use a wheelchair.

(B) Identify The Fears Within The Fear

I feared dogs, but big dogs scared me more than small dogs. Size mattered, yet not always. Petting a large dog through a fence would be easier than play-wrestling with a tiny one in its backyard, and looking at a picture of several Great Danes would be easier than hearing two nearby yapping toy poodles. So, type of activity and proximity mattered, too, and so did number depending on circumstance. The absolutely scariest doggie situation would be being chased by a large growling salivating beast.

Let's return to the aversion to being in a wheelchair in public. Specifically, what would be the most discomforting situation involving a wheelchair at the mall? Suppose it is being in a clothes store and asking the salesperson where the try-on rooms are. Now think about other situations, less upsetting but related or leading to that worst one. Write them down on separate cards or use your computer; don't worry about which scene in this list is more upsetting than another in this list—for now.

Overcoming Disabilities despair

Worst situation:

Being in a wheelchair and asking the salesperson in the clothes store where to try on the merchandise selected.

Other situations:

- Driving to the mall with the wheelchair in the trunk
- Sitting alone at home thinking about being at the mall in a wheelchair
- Being seen by coworkers while wheeling around the mall
- Being seen by spouse's coworkers while wheeling around the mall
- Being seen by strangers while wheeling around the mall
- Spending one hour in the mall in a wheelchair
- Spending 20 minutes in the mall in a wheelchair
- Entering a clothes store in a wheelchair and looking at the merchandise
- Spending the entire morning in the mall in a wheelchair
- Spending the entire day in the mall in a wheelchair
- While in wheelchair, purchasing an item in a clothes store
- While in a wheelchair, asking the salesperson in the clothes store for help

(C) Rank Order The Fear Situations

Categorize the situations into mildly disturbing, moderately disturbing, and very disturbing. Then, within each category, rank each situation from one (low discomfort) to 10 (high discomfort). If while doing this you think of new situations, fit them in. Your first attempt, perhaps your final ordering, might look like this:

Mildly disturbing:

1) Sitting alone at home thinking about being at mall in a wheelchair

2) Driving to the mall with the wheelchair in the trunk

Moderately disturbing:

1) Spending 20 minutes in the mall in a wheelchair

2) Spending one hour in the mall in a wheelchair

3) Being seen by strangers while wheeling around the mall

4) Being seen by spouse's coworkers while wheeling around the mall

Severely disturbing:

5) Being seen by coworkers while wheeling around the mall

6) Spending the entire morning in the mall in a wheelchair

7) Spending the entire day in the mall in a wheelchair

8) Entering a clothes store in a wheelchair and looking at the merchandise

9) While in a wheelchair, asking the salesperson in the clothes store for help

10) While in wheelchair, purchasing an item in a clothes store

11) While in a wheelchair, asking the salesperson in the clothes store where to try on the merchandise selected.

(D) Devour The Fear

You have two choices in how you consume it: all at once or piece-by-piece. The "all at once" method, called flooding, means tackling your worst fear right from the start—no build up to it; you wheel into the store and ask the salesperson where to try on the clothes you've selected. Flooding works sometimes, but I don't recommend it. Too scary; occasionally it overwhelms you. I favor the "piece-by-piece" strategy. It starts with the least fearful situation and inches-up to the most; this slower, gentler, overtime way works well, especially when combined with Dr. Edmund Bourne's sequence of exposure, retreat, recover, repeat, described in his, *The anxiety & phobia workbook.*

Begin with the first situation in the mildly disturbing category. So, sit alone in your living room and think about being at the mall in a wheelchair. Keep imagining until comfortable or at least until discomfort becomes manageable. Then, when convenient, go to situation two in that category—yes, take a drive to the mall with the wheelchair in your trunk. Continue with this exposure phase until you have dealt with all situations in all categories. Always go from easiest to hardest—situation by situation, category by category.

The anxiety or discomfort you feel in some situations may take only a few minutes to vanquish, whereas in others it may take much longer. Be patient, be determined. Stick to it. Practice daily. As you work to conquer the fears within the fear, it's okay to feel (as Bourne suggests) somewhat anxious, butterflies-in-the-stomach-anxious, yet still in control. But, as he cautions, stop the procedure when control seems like it's vanishing; retreat until better.

Then when recovered—and practicing relaxation will speed recovery—go back at it (repeat the exposure). Keep doing the exposure, retreat, recover, repeat dance until discomfort vanishes altogether or becomes tolerable, and you're free enough from whatever has been holding you back.

To motivate yourself to do these procedures and stick to them, consider contracting with yourself (see above). Consider also including a friend or loved-one to join with you in working through the discomforting situations. Go to the mall with somebody, maybe let her push the wheelchair. Make sure you choose a trustworthy, reliable, upbeat soul and not a judge, blamer, or shamer. And whether going it alone or not, encourage yourself with confidence-building thoughts, such as:

I know if I face my fear, I'll get free of it

If things get too upsetting, I can stop until I feel better

I'm the boss of this

Inch- by-inch — no hurry, I can handle this.

A final word. Tenacity. When using CBT tools like relaxation or exposure, don't expect immediate change. Practice, practice, practice.

LAST WORD:

Perhaps An In-VA-lid But Never In-VAL-id

I hope you have found this book helpful, see its possibilities in continuing to help you, and will keep using it when disability assumptions drag you down. Dispute the assumptions declaring your future hopeless, your present joyless, and you helpless, ugly, or worthless. Fail to do so, and you risk making life far less than it could be, far less than it should be. As you hone the skills for listening to and disputing misery-generating thoughts, watch out for the disabilities-mind-set, that inner voice saying:

I am desperate. You, understandably, might be desperate, but keep desperation from clouding discernment. Remain skeptical of miracle-like remedies backed up only by testimonials, not scientific data. Resist the temptation to buy and try them, for they will more often disappoint and possibly harm than help.

I am my disability. Don't let your disability define you and allow prejudgments about what your disability permits and prevents to contaminate decisions about what you can and cannot do. Don't let your disability define you and put limits on what you can accomplish, on who you are, or on who you can be.

I am disabled, so of course I'm depressed. Having disabilities is no picnic, but it's not the end of the world either. If depressed, take steps to not be. Mope less to cope more.

I am disabled, so I can't.... Yes you can. Surprise yourself with how often you can. A special friend sat across from me in our living room as I struggled to remove my leg brace. I had just returned from the University and was trying to get comfortable before dinner. Seeing how tired I was and wanting to help, she stood up, walked the few paces towards me, and said kindly, "I'll do it. Just sit back." Because I value her so much, I did not want to thwart her good intentions. Nonetheless, I declined the offer. Not only do I need to feel independent, but also I need to realize it's likely neither she nor anyone else will be there next time. Okay, one exception wouldn't kill me, but I hold good practices dear and try to repeat them whenever I can. Use it or lose it faster is my mantra, and one I recommend to all with disabilities. Be stubborn.

BUT NOT STUPID. As Emerson said, "A foolish consistency is the hobgoblin of little minds." Use in order not to lose faster makes sense, but eagerly embracing sound principles must not mutate into blindly obeying them.

Several years ago my routine after driving to work was to carefully to lift my walker from the trunk and push-roll to my nearby office, but one day this routine was interrupted. My walker was jammed in the trunk. So, I yanked it upward quite forcibly. Tug one rocked me backward, but luckily I caught myself and remained vertical. I wanted to try tug two and, if necessary, to keep tugging until succeeding — the stubborn part of me. The not wanting to be stupid part of me, however, envisioned yours truly on the ground in pain. Unlikely? Likely? Possibly? I decided not to find out. So, I asked the first person walking by to lend a hand. Maybe I didn't need to, but why chance it. Admittedly, realizing the difference between stubborn and stupid isn't always easy.

Accept being disabled. Living with disabilities can make you miserable, if because of what you tell yourself you let it. Try to not let it. Tell yourself, okay I am disabled but I'll handle it, take what comes, do what I must. So, if necessary adjust your external environment for your physical well-being and modify your internal environment for your psychological well-being. Apropos of the latter, think better to prevent disability assumptions that fuel fear, siphon power, and diminish life from taking over and pushing you deep into despair.

And, think clearly to prevent yourself from presuming that an incapacity of limb somehow signifies an inferiority of person, an

Overcoming Disabilities despair

absurd presumption to say the least but one held too often by too many disabled men and women. As my erudite friend and colleague, Dr. Fred Marcuse, himself disabled after a vicious automobile accident, would so pithily remark, "Invalid (in-va-lid) isn't invalid (in-val-id)."

> "One Person Plus One Wheelchair Patron"

[Sign on elevator for the disabled at popular local entertainment spot]

Overcoming Disabilities despair

REFERENCES

American Psychiatric Association. Diagnostics and statistics manual of the American Psychiatric Association fourth edition (1994). Washington, D.C.: American Psychiatric Association.

Beck, A.T., Rush , A.J., Shaw, B.F., & Emery, G. (1979).Cognitive therapy of depression. New York: Guilford.

.Bootzin, R. (1977) Behavioral treatment of insomnia: a clinician's guide and self-management techniques for controlling insomnia. New York: Audiocassette Programs.

Bourne, E.J. The anxiety & phobia workbook (1995). Oakland: New Harbinger Publications, Inc.

Burns, D.D. (1989). The feeling good handbook. Ontario: Penguin Books (Plume).

Covey, S.R. The 7 habits of highly effective people (1989). New York: Simon & Schuster.

Dawodu, S.T. Spinal Cord Injury - Definition, Epidemiology, Pathophysiology Updated: Mar 30, 2009

http://emedicine.medscape.com/article/322480-overview

Grand, L. C.(2000). The marriage & family presentation guide. New York: John Wiley & Sons, Inc.

Jacobson, E. (1929). Progressive relaxation. Chicago: University of Chicago Press.

Leahy, R. & Holland S. (2000). Treatment plans and interventions for depression and anxiety disorders New York: Guilford.

Multiple Sclerosis Council, Fatigue and multiple sclerosis: evidence-based management strategies for fatigue in multiple sclerosis (1998). (For a copy of this report, write the PARALYZED VETERANS OF

AMERICA, 801 18th Street, N. W., Washington D.C. 20006-3517).

Polman, P. Drug treatment of multiple sclerosis, BMJ Vitdehaag, 2001, 321, 490-494.

Schapiro, R. What is MS, International MS Support Group, 2001.(www. msnews.org/fair2.shtml).

Scholcket, S. Bertelson, A., & Lacks, P. (1988). Is sleep hygiene a sufficient treatment for sleep-maintenance insomnia? Behavior therapy, 19, 183-190.

Thomas, G. (1986), Leader effectiveness training New York: Bantam Doubleday Dell.

APPENDIX 1

LeBOW ASSUMPTIONS OF DISABILITY INVENTORY

THIS INVENTORY IS PRIMARILY FOR THOSE WHO ARE DISABLED, ESPECIALLY THOSE DISABLED TO THE EXTENT THEY REQUIRE A CANE, WALKER, OR WHEELCHAIR.

DESCRIPTION AND INSTRUCTIONS:

The inventory comprises 31 statements that reflect your opinions about your being disabled. Each asks you to judge, from "Not At All" to "A Lot," the extent you agree with the statement. Total scores will vary from 0 (if you answered "Not At All" to each of them) to 93 (if you answered "A Lot" to each of them). The lower your total score the better, meaning the greater your freedom from debilitating disability assumptions.

Take the inventory now and retake it periodically as you learn to question and challenge the misery-generating disability assumptions depressing you. By retaking it as you try out the book's procedures, you'll be able to judge (as your total score lowers) how much you are improving. As well, you'll be able to judge, as regards each particular statement, how your ratings change. Your objective is to move from individual statement-ratings of 3 and 2 ("A Lot" and "Moderately") to those of 1 and 0 ("Somewhat" and "Not At All"). A recording sheet for your benefit follows the questionnaire.

1. Because I am disabled, I've lost most chances to enjoy life. To what extent do you agree?

0 (Not At All) 1 (Somewhat) 2 (Moderately) 3 (A Lot)

2. Because I am disabled, I no longer have anything to offer others. To what extent do you agree?

0 (Not At All) 1 (Somewhat) 2 (Moderately) 3 (A Lot)

3. Because I am disabled, I burden friends. To what extent do you agree?

0 (Not At All) 1 (Somewhat) 2 (Moderately) 3 (A Lot)

4. Because I am disabled, others who are not disabled are uncomfortable around me. To what extent do you agree?

0 (Not At All) 1 (Somewhat) 2 (Moderately) 3 (A Lot)

5. Because I am disabled, I am less worthy. To what extent do you agree?

0 (Not At All) 1 (Somewhat) 2 (Moderately) 3 (A Lot)

6. Because I am disabled, I have less to offer others. To what extent do you agree?

0 (Not At All) 1 (Somewhat) 2 (Moderately) 3 (A Lot)

7. Because I am disabled, I am less socially appealing. To what extent do you agree?

0 (Not At All) 1 (Somewhat) 2 (Moderately) 3 (A Lot)

8. Others don't accept me as their equal now that I am disabled. To what extent do you agree.

0 (Not At All) 1 (Somewhat) 2 (Moderately) 3 (A Lot)

9. Because I am disabled, all the changes in my life will be negative. To what extent do you agree?

0 (Not At All) 1 (Somewhat) 2 (Moderately) 3 (A Lot)

10. Because I am disabled, I'm easier to ignore. To what extent do you agree?

0 (Not At All) 1 (Somewhat) 2 (Moderately) 3 (A Lot)

11. Because I am disabled, I'm ugly. To what extent do you agree?

0 (Not At All) 1 (Somewhat) 2 (Moderately) 3 (A Lot)

12. Because I am disabled, there is little I can do about the problems facing me. To what extent you agree?

0 (Not At All) 1 (Somewhat) 2 (Moderately) 3 (A Lot)

13. Because I am disabled, I have little or no chance of doing something in the future I can be proud of. To what extent do you agree?

0 (Not At All) 1 (Somewhat) 2 (Moderately) 3 (A Lot)

14. Because I am disabled. To what extent do you agree?

0 (Not At All) 1 (Somewhat) 2 (Moderately) 3 (A Lot)

15. Because I am disabled, most of the future changes in my life will likely be negative. To what extent do you agree?

0 (Not At All) 1 (Somewhat) 2 (Moderately) 3 (A Lot)

16. Because I am disabled, I'm no longer able to do the important things. To what extent do you agree?

0 (Not At All) 1 (Somewhat) 2 (Moderately) 3 (A Lot)

17. Because I am disabled, most others pity me. To what extent do you agree?

0 (Not At All) 1 (Somewhat) 2 (Moderately) 3 (A Lot)

18. Because I am disabled, my future looks hopeless. To what extent do you agree?

0 (Not At All) 1 (Somewhat) 2 (Moderately) 3 (A Lot)

19. Because I am disabled, I burden my family. To what extent do you agree?

0 (Not At All) 1 (Somewhat) 2 (Moderately) 3 (A Lot)

20. Because I am disabled, life no longer is fun and exciting. To what extent do you agree?

0 (Not At All) 1 (Somewhat) 2 (Moderately) 3 (A Lot)

21. Now that I am disabled, I am vulnerable. To what extent do you agree?

0 (Not At All) 1 (Somewhat) 2 (Moderately) 3 (A Lot)

22. If I can't do as much as I used to, I'm not as worthy as I once was. To what extent do you agree?

0 (Not At All) 1 (Somewhat) 2 (Moderately) 3 (A Lot)

23. Because I am disabled, I'm less appealing sexually. To what extent do you agree?

0 (Not At All) 1 (Somewhat) 2 (Moderately) 3 (A Lot)

24. Because I am disabled, I have little chance in the future of excelling. To what extent do you agree?

0 (Not At All) 1 (Somewhat) 2 (Moderately) 3 (A Lot)

25. To many others, my disability is like a neon sign flashing avoid me. To what extent do you agree?

0 (Not At All) 1 (Somewhat) 2 (Moderately) 3 (A Lot)

26. Because I am disabled, I've lost all chances to enjoy life. To what extent do you agree?

0 (Not At All) 1 (Somewhat) 2 (Moderately) 3 (A Lot)

27. Because I am disabled, I have much less to offer others. To what extent do you agree?

0 (Not At All) 1 (Somewhat) 2 (Moderately) 3 (A Lot)

28. Because I am disabled, all future changes in my life will likely be negative. To what extent do you agree?

0 (Not At All) 1 (Somewhat) 2 (Moderately) 3 (A Lot)

29. Because I am disabled, more people than ever before do not wish to be around me. To what extent do you agree?

0 (Not At All) 1 (Somewhat) 2 (Moderately) 3 (A Lot)

30. There is little I can do about the problems my being disabled causes me. To what extent do you agree?

0 (Not At All) 1 (Somewhat) 2 (Moderately) 3 (A Lot)

31. Because I am disabled, I'm unappealing sexually. To what extent do you agree?

0 (Not At All) 1 (Somewhat) 2 (Moderately) 3 (A Lot)

TOTAL SCORE=

Overcoming Disabilities despair

ANSWER SHEET Record your answers to the inventory each time you take it by putting a 0(not at all), 1(somewhat), 2(moderately), or 3(a lot) in the space to the right of the numbers, each of which represents one of the 31 statements. Then, total your score (T) and indicate the date (D).

	time1	time 2	time 3	time 4
1				
2				
3				
4				
5				
6				
7				
8				
9				
10				
11				
12				
13				
14				
15				

Overcoming Disabilities despair

16				
17				
18				
19				
20				
21				
22				
23				
24				
25				
26				
26				
27				
29				
30				
31				
Total				
Date				

Overcoming Disabilities despair

APPENDIX 2

Algorithm: Nine Steps for Talking Away What's Getting You Down

STEP 1 DESCRIBE WHAT HAPPENED THAT UPSET YOU

Something upset you. Write down what. Possibly nothing specific you can name took place other than just thinking of things — daydreams, recollections, worries about what's to come — and your depressed mood seems with worsen or harden; detail your thoughts.

STEP 2 NAME AND RATE YOUR NEGATIVE FEELINGS

Write down your feelings - name them - and rate how strongly from 1 (hardly at all) to 100 (extremely) you feel them

STEP 3. IDENTIFY EACH MISERY-GENERATING ASSUMPTION TRIGGERED

Ask yourself why you feel the way you feel. To answer, try to recover the thoughts you had when the situation that upset you happened — replay your inner voice . From those thoughts search for each misery-making assumption triggered. Do each assumption separately.

List Your Disabling Thoughts & Search for the Underlying Disability Assumption and from the list of possibilities below:

Possible Disability Assumptions:

1) If I'm disabled, my worth is diminished, and there's nothing I can do about it

2) If I'm disabled, I can never be happy again, and there's nothing I can do about it

3) If I'm disabled, I look ugly, and there's nothing I

can do about it

4) If I'm disabled, I'm helpless, and there's nothing I can do about it

5) If I'm disabled, I have no hope for the future, and there's nothing I can do about it

State the Disability Assumption You Identify:

STEP 4. RATE HOW MUCH YOU AGREE THAT THE ASSUMPTION IDENTIFIED IS TRUE

For each assumption triggered, rate to what extent you agree that it is true: [0.Not at all, 1.Somewhat, 2.Moderately 3. A Lot]

STEP 5. DISPUTE BY QUESTIONING THE ASSUMPTION IDENTIFIED

Dispute the assumption by questioning its value, logic, fairness, evidence, or

accuracy, or all these qualities using one or more over the 10 questions in the list below. Think hard.

Possible Questions To Ask:

1) What Are The Pluses of Accepting And Those of Rejecting The Assumption?

2) Would I Say it to Someone Else?

3) How Do I Figure?

4) Am I Thinking Rigidly?

5) Am I Labeling?

6) What Are The Exceptions (Search for Exceptions)?

7) Am I Fortune-telling?

8) Am I Catastrophizing?

9) Am I Letting My Feelings Be My Reality?

10) What Would a High-priced Lawyer Say?

Actual Questions Asked:

STEP 6 DISPUTE BY CHALLENGING THE ASSUMPTION IDENTIFIED

Dispute the assumption by challenging behaviorally the part that says, "and there's nothing I can do about it." Make a challenge to that part using one or more of the six challenges in the list below. Refute or cast reasonable doubt on the assumption, by doing something constructive.

Possible Challenges to Make:

1) Challenge by Assertiveness

2) Challenge by Activation

3) Challenge by Problem-solving

4) Challenge by Contracting

5) Challenge by Relaxation

6) Challenge by Exposure

Actual Challenges Made:

STEP 7. REAPPRAISE

Devise a fairer, more helpful way of looking at whatever triggered— incidents, comments, recollections, etc.—the nasty assumption identified. Compare your thinking now with your thinking then. Look at what you said in step three. What would you say now? You may have to think about that for a few days or weeks first.

STEP 8. CONSIDER AGAIN THE MISERY-GENERATING ASSUMPTION IDENTIFIED AND RE-RATE HOW MUCH YOU AGREE THAT IT IS TRUE

What do you now say after having questioned and challenged the assumption and reappraised the events triggering it? Apply the scale used in step 4 and compare your responses then with those now.

Possible ratings:

0. Not at all

1. Somewhat

2. Moderately

3. A Lot

Previous rating:

Current rating:

STEP 9. RE-RATE THE STRENGTH OF THE EMOTIONS YOU NAMED PREVIOUSLY

As in step 2, rate from 1 to 100 the degree you feel each emotion. Compare your ratings now with those made before and note the difference, if any.

Previous rating:

Current rating:

APPENDIX 3

Activity Baseline Form

Day Date

Instructions: For each interval write what you did and how pleasurable each activity was. Rate from zero to ten (e.g., 0=no pleasure, 5=moderately pleasurable, 10= the most pleasure you can think of). Place this number immediately after the activity. Also, rate how much of a mastery feeling (sense of achievement, competency, effectiveness, independence) doing it gave you from 0-10 (0=no mastery, 5=a moderate amount, 10= the most you can imagine). Place this number after the pleasure rating (e.g., watching two hours of morning television, 2/0).

7-10am

After 10am-1pm

After 1pm-4pm

After 4pm-7pm

After 7pm-10pm

After 11pm-wake-up

Overcoming Disabilities despair

APPENDIX 4

Activities Planned and Completed Form

Day Date Instructions: For each interval write what you plan to do in the Planned column and complete in the Completed column. For each planned activity predict how pleasurable it will be from zero to ten (e.g., 0=no pleasure, 5=moderately pleasurable, 10= the most pleasure you can think of). Place this number immediately after the planned activity. Also, predict how much of a mastery feeling (sense of achievement, competency, effectiveness, independence) doing it will give from 0-10 (0=no mastery, 5=a moderate amount, 10= the most you can imagine). Place this number after the pleasure rating (e.g., exercising 20 minutes, 3/2). Make the same two ratings for the activity, after having done it, in the Completed column (e.g., exercising 20 minutes, 4/5) — the pleasure and mastery experience. For activities that occupy more than one interval, just note the particulars on the form by the entry. Also, note planned activities not completed

Overcoming Disabilities despair

7-10am

Planned							Completed

After 10am-1pm

Planned							Completed

After 1pm-4pm

Planned							Completed

After 4pm-7pm

Planned							Completed

After 7pm-11pm

Planned							Completed

After 11pm-wake-up

Planned							Completed

INDEX

Activation
    baseline, sample 48
    challenges 46
    how to plan 48, 49
    planned completed, sample
   50
    pleasure, mastery............47
    Stoppers 51
Activities Planned and Completed Form (blank) ...135
Algorithm
    applicability 5, 88
    arguing against propositions
   35
    disability assumptions (see Disability Assumptions
Ally Koulack-Wilson & stroke 55
Amantadine and Pemoline ...93
Anti-fatigue" Medicines.........93
Anxiety & phobia workbook 113
Assertiveness .. 30, 46, 61, 74, 84, 105, 106, 131
assumptions
    productive 8-9
    silent 8
Assumptions, disability (see Disability Assumptions)
Assumptions, dysfunctional
    samples 8-10
Attila the Hun..........................1
Autoimmune diseases..........69
Baseline form (blank form) 133
Beck, Aaron 5, 8, 119
Body mass index (BMI) 55
Bootzin, Richard 96, 119
booze 97
Bourne, Edmund 113
brainstorming.......................77
breath-counting 109

breath-holding.................... 108
breathing rhythmically........ 108
bribery................................ 108
Burns, David 5, 8
caffeine 97
Cases
    Ally.................55-62 , 66, 67
    David 37
    Julie 21-34, 53-69
    Matthias..................... 69-88
cervical, thoracic, lumbar..... 38
Challenges
    activation (see also Activation) .... I 46-51, 106
    assertiveness.... 30-31, 105
    contracting (see also Contract) ... 61-64 ,107-108
    exposure (see also Exposure).............. 109-114
    problem-solving...................
    .... 75-76, 84-86, 106-107
    relaxation...................... 108
Changing time zones........... 94
Chronic progressive multiple sclerosis.............................. 2
Cognitive Behavior Therapy (CBT) .... 5, 6 ,89, 103, 114
Cognitive therapy of depression
.... 8
Contract 61- 64
    Do's, Don'ts, Consequences 63
    tips on writing 64- 65
Covey, Stephen 5
David Perry & SCI............. 37
demyelinating...................... 22
depositing inflammatory cells 69
Diaphragm breathing 109
Disabilities despair 5, 13, 21 ,22, 38, 53, 88

Disabilities-mind-set 115
Disability Assumptions
    challenging (see Challenges)described 10-12
    disability diminishes worth ... 10, 21-35
    disability ends happiness 11, 37- 53 ....
    disability means helpless 11, 69-77
    disability means hopeless 12, 79 -89
    disability means ugly number 11, 55- 67
    identifying 25, 39, 58, 67, 80
    questioning (see Questions)
    re-rating feelings 32, 52, 67, 77, 88
    re-rating truth of 32, 52, 67,77, 87
    reappraising 32, 51, 66 , 76, 87
Disability Fallout
    fatigue 91, 93
    relating 98-102
    sleep 93-98
Disability fatigue
    activate, Don't Over-activate 91
    cool 92
    good sleep 93
    medicines 93
    nap..................................92
    relax 93
Disability inventory.......... 14-18
    scoring form 19-20
DSM 4 94
Ellis, Albert 5
Emerson, Ralph Waldo 116
emotional reasoning 12, 60, 84, 105
Energy effectiveness 92
Exposure 109-114
confidence building thoughts 113-114
devour the fear 112-113
Flooding vs. piece by piece 112-113
identify fear................... 110
identify fears within the fear 110
rank order fears............ 111
exposure, retreat, recover, repeat 113
Fatigue.......................... 91-93
Feeling good handbook .. 8, 25
Fields, WC 2
Hawking, Stephen 82
Hercules Poirot 13
Holland, Stephen . 96, 108, 109
Grand, Laurie Cope ... 100, 119
Insulin-dependent-diabetes-mellitus(IDDM) 56
in-va-lid isn't in-val-id 117
Jacobson, Edmund.... 108, 119
lapse vs. relapse................. 35
Leahy, Robert 96, 108, 109
Listening, empathically 101-102
Lyme's disease 101
Macrophages 23
Marcuse, Fred................. 117
Marriage& Family Presentation Guide 100
Melatonin 94
Modafinil (Alertec)................ 93
Multiple sclerosis 2, 9, 12, 21, 91, 93, 108, 109, 119, 120
Multiple Sclerosis Council of America 91, 119
Myelin....................... 22, 23, 69
Narcolepsy 93
Non-insulin-dependent-diabetes-mellitus(NIDDM) .. 56
Obstructive sleep apnea...... 95
One Person Plus One Wheelchair Patron (sign)... 118

orthotic device 57
Overactivate 91, 92
Porter, Bill................................8
Problem solving 30, 46, 61, 74, 75, 84, 106, 131
Progressive Relaxation 108
quadriplegia,........................ 38
Questions
    catastrophizing 82, 104
    accepting or rejecting assumptions 28, 45, 83, 103
    emotional reasoning .60, 84, 105
    exceptions 104
    fairness (double standard) 29, 61, 83, 103
    fortune-telling73, 81-82, 104
    high-priced lawyer ...41, 105
    how do you figure (evidence, logic) 29-30, 104
    labeling 73, 104
    thinking rigidly ... 60, 74, 104
rapid eye movement (REM) .94
Reeve, Christopher 82
Relating 98-102
Relaxation
    Breath-holding 108-109
    breath counting..............109
    breathing rhythmically....108
    diaphragm breathing 109
Rewards 107-108
Rheumatoid arthritis (RA)..5, 9, 12, 69, 108
rheumatoid nodules..............69
Ritalin...................................93
Scholcket, S 96, 120
Segun T. Dawodu 38, 119
7 habits of highly effective people......................................5
Sjögren's syndrome..............69
Sleep and sleep troubles 93-95
Sleep stages........................94
Solving problems together 101

Spinal cord 37-38, 108
Stimulus control 95-96
Stroke 57, 67
Synovial fluid........................ 69
T(5)fifth thoracic vertebrae37,38
Talking turn-offs..............98-99
Talking turn-ons........... 99-102
tetraplegia 38
Treatment Plans and Interventions for Depression and Anxiety disorders 108
Type I diabetes 56
Type II diabetes 55, 56, 57
Vertical arrow technique 25

Science & Humanities Press

Publishes fine books under the imprints:
- Science & Humanities Press
- BeachHouse Books
- MacroPrint Books
- Heuristic Books
- Early Editions Books

Educators & Seniors Discount Policy

To encourage use of our books for education, educators can purchase three or more books (mixed titles) on our standard discount schedule for resellers. See **sciencehumanitiespress.com/educator/educator.html** for more detail.

Science & Humanities Press
PO Box 7151
Chesterfield MO 63006-7151
636-394-4950

Printed in Great Britain
by Amazon.co.uk, Ltd.,
Marston Gate.